Shoulder Rehabilitation

Editor

THOMAS (QUIN) THROCKMORTON

PHYSICAL MEDICINE AND REHABILITATION CLINICS OF NORTH AMERICA

www.pmr.theclinics.com

Consulting Editor
SANTOS F. MARTINEZ

May 2023 • Volume 34 • Number 2

ELSEVIER

1600 John F. Kennedy Boulevard ● Suite 1800 ● Philadelphia, Pennsylvania, 19103-2899

http://www.theclinics.com

PHYSICAL MEDICINE AND REHABILITATION CLINICS OF NORTH AMERICA Volume 34, Number 2
May 2023 ISSN 1047-9651, 978-0-323-96060-1

Editor: Megan Ashdown
Developmental Editor: Diana Grace Ang

Reprints. For copies of 100 or more of articles in this publication, please contact the Commercial Reprints Department, Elsevier Inc., 360 Park Avenue South, New York, NY 10010-1710. Tel.: 212-633-3874; Fax: 212-633-3820; E-mail: reprints@elsevier.com.

Physical Medicine and Rehabilitation Clinics of North America (ISSN 1047-9651) is published quarterly by Elsevier Inc., 360 Park Avenue South, New York, NY 10010-1710. Months of issue are February, May, August, and November. Business and Editorial Offices: 1600 John F. Kennedy Blvd., Suite 1800, Philadelphia, PA 19103-2899. Customer Service Office: 3251 Riverport Lane, Maryland Heights, MO 63043. Periodicals postage paid at New York, NY and additional mailing offices. Subscription price per year is $342.00 (US individuals), $722.00 (US institutions), $100.00 (US students), $388.00 (Canadian individuals), $950.00 (Canadian institutions), $100.00 (Canadian students), $491.00 (foreign individuals), $950.00 (foreign institutions), and $210.00 (foreign students). Foreign air speed delivery is included in all *Clinics* subscription prices. All prices are subject to change without notice. **POSTMASTER:** Send address changes to *Physical Medicine and Rehabilitation Clinics of North America*, Customer Service Office: Elsevier Health Sciences Division, Subscription Customer Service, 3251 Riverport Lane, Maryland Heights, MO 63043. **Customer Service: 1-800-654-2452 (US). From outside of the United States, call 314-447-8871. Fax: 314-447-8029. E-mail: JournalsCustomerService-usa@elsevier.com (for print support); JournalsOnlineSupport-usa@elsevier.com (for online support).**

Physical Medicine and Rehabilitation Clinics of North America is indexed in *Excerpta Medica, MEDLINE/PubMed (Index Medicus), Cinahl,* and *Cumulative Index to Nursing and Allied Health Literature.*

Contributors

CONSULTING EDITOR

SANTOS F. MARTINEZ, MD, MS
Assistant Professor, Department of Orthopaedic Surgery and Biomedical Engineering,
University of Tennessee College of Medicine, Memphis, Tennessee

EDITOR

THOMAS (QUIN) THROCKMORTON, MD
Professor, Shoulder and Elbow Surgery, University of Tennessee-Campbell Clinic,
Department of Orthopaedic Surgery, Memphis, Tennessee

AUTHORS

ABDULAZIZ F. AHMED, MD
Department of Orthopedic Surgery, Massachusetts General Hospital, Harvard Medical
School, Boston, Massachusetts

WILLIAM R. AIBINDER, MD
Clinical Assistant Professor, Department of Orthopaedic Surgery, University of Michigan,
Ann Arbor, Michigan

ALYSSA D. ALTHOFF, MD
Department of Orthopaedic Surgery, University of Virginia, Charlottesville, Virginia

W. BEN KIBLER, MD
Shoulder Center of Kentucky, Lexington Clinic, Lexington, Kentucky

STEPHEN BROCKMEIER, MD
Department of Orthopaedic Surgery, University of Virginia, Charlottesville, Virginia

TYLER J. BROLIN, MD
The University of Tennessee Health Science Center-Campbell Clinic, Memphis Tennessee

COLBY BRUNETTE, BS
Department of Orthopaedic Surgery, University of Virginia, Charlottesville, Virginia

PETER CHALMERS, MD
Instructor, Department of Shoulder and Elbow Surgery, University of Utah, Salt Lake City,
Utah

ROBIN CROMWELL, PT
Department of Physical Therapy, Lexington Clinic, Lexington, Kentucky

REBECCA N. DICKINSON, PT, DPT, OCS
Vanderbilt Orthopedics Nashville, Nashville, Tennessee

BASSEM T. ELHASSAN, MD
Co-Chief, MGH Shoulder Service, Department of Orthopedic Surgery, Massachusetts General Hospital, Professor of Orthopedic Surgery, Harvard Medical School, Boston, Massachusetts

BRANDON J. ERICKSON, MD
Rothman Orthopaedic Institute, Assistant Professor, Department of Orthopaedic Surgery, Sidney Kimmel Medical College, Thomas Jefferson University, NYU Grossman School of Medicine, New York University, New York, New York

RACHEL M. FRANK, MD
Department of Orthopedic Surgery, University of Colorado School of Medicine, Aurora, Colorado

GRANT E. GARRIGUES, MD
Department of Orthopaedic Surgery, Rush University Medical Center, Midwest Orthopaedics at Rush, Chicago, Illinois

REUBEN GOBEZIE, MD
Assistant Professor, Cleveland Shoulder Institute, Beachwood, Ohio

JEFFREY R. HILL, MD
Orthopedic Surgery Shoulder Fellow, Department of Orthopaedic Surgery, Washington University, St Louis, Missouri

EVAN H. HOROWITZ, MD
Resident Physician, Department of Orthopaedic Surgery and Rehabilitation Medicine, SUNY Downstate Health Sciences University, Brooklyn, New York

JAY D. KEENER, MD, PT
Professor, Department of Orthopaedic Surgery, Washington University, St Louis, Missouri

JOHN E. KUHN, MS, MD
Kenneth D. Schermerhorn Professor of Orthopaedics, Vanderbilt Orthopedics Nashville, Nashville, Tennessee

NELS LEAFBLAD, MD
Fellow, Department of Sports Medicine, University of Utah, Salt Lake City, Utah

JOHN WILLIAM LOCKHART, PT, DPT
Department of Physical Therapy, Lexington Clinic, Lexington, Kentucky

RYAN LOHRE, MD
Department of Orthopedic Surgery, Massachusetts General Hospital, Harvard Medical School, Boston, Massachusetts

TIMOTHY P. MCCARTHY, MD
Department of Orthopedic Surgery, University of Colorado Medical Center, Aurora, Colorado

MARIANO E. MENENDEZ, MD
Oregon Shoulder Institute at Southern Oregon Orthopedics, Medford, Oregon

JOSH MIZELS, MD
Resident, Department of Orthopaedic Surgery, University of Utah, Salt Lake City, Utah

JOHN MOTLEY, PT, ATC, CSCS
Staff Physical Therapist, Barnes Jewish West County Hospital

ANAND M. MURTHI, MD
Department of Orthopaedics, MedStar Union Memorial Hospital, Baltimore, Maryland

WILLIAM POLIO, MD
The University of Tennessee Health Science Center-Campbell Clinic, Memphis
Tennessee

AARON SCIASCIA, PhD, ATC, PES, SMTC, FNAP
Institute for Clinical Outcomes and Research, Lexington Clinic, Lexington, Kentucky

YOUSEF SHISHANI, MD
Assistant Professor, Cleveland Shoulder Institute, Beachwood, Ohio

DANIEL J. STOKES, MD
Department of Orthopedic Surgery, University of Colorado School of Medicine, Aurora,
Colorado

SULEIMAN Y. SUDAH, MD
Department of Orthopedics, Monmouth Medical Center, Long Branch, New Jersey

TAYLOR SWANSEN, MD
Department of Orthopaedics, MedStar Union Memorial Hospital, Baltimore, Maryland

ROBERT TASHJIAN, MD
Professor, Department of Shoulder and Elbow Surgery, University of Utah, Salt Lake City,
Utah

MELISSA A. WRIGHT, MD
Department of Orthopaedics, MedStar Union Memorial Hospital, Baltimore, Maryland

Contents

advances in progress-based steps during 24 weeks. The rehabilitation process aims to balance healing of the tendon repair and the risk of post-operative stiffness.

The long head of the biceps and superior labrum should be evaluated as an interdependent functional unit. A focused patient history and physical examination including multiple provocative tests should be performed alongside advanced imaging studies to obtain an accurate diagnosis. Nonoperative treatment modalities including nonsteroidal anti-inflammatory drugs, glucocorticoid injections, and a standardized physical therapy regimen should be exhausted before operative intervention. Significant improvements in pain, functional outcomes, and quality of life are achieved in patients treated nonoperatively. Although these outcomes are less consistent for overhead athletes, return to play and performance metrics seem comparable to those who undergo surgery.

The 4-phase rehabilitation protocol outlined in this article provides a comprehensive 26-week program to return patients with superior labrum anterior posterior repairs to their preinjury states. It is guided by the principle of gradual return to preinjury function while preserving the integrity of the surgical repair. Objective criteria are present at the conclusion of each phase to ensure patients are progressing appropriately. The goal is to allow patients to return to their previous functional ability in their sport-specific or occupational-specific training.

Shoulder instability is the separation of the humeral head from the glenoid. Injury to the static and dynamic stabilizers can result in instability. Anterior shoulder instability is the predominant form of instability. It is usually a result of trauma. Posterior shoulder instability often presents with an insidious onset of pain. Multidirectional instability of the shoulder is symptomatic laxity in more than one plane of motion. The primary goal of rehabilitation is to restore pain-free mobility, strength, and functioning. Rehabilitation implements range of motion and strengthening exercises to restore proprioceptive control and scapular kinematics.

Shoulder instability can occur in any direction and presents across a broad spectrum including traumatic dislocations, repetitive microinstability events or subluxations, and global joint laxity. The development of pain, functional decline, and articular pathologic condition is a multifaceted process that is influenced by the underlying bony morphology, biology of the surrounding soft tissue structures, dynamic coordination of the periscapular musculature, and patient factors such as age, activity level, and associated injuries. This article will focus on the younger, active patient with instability due to deficiencies in the capsulolabral complex and dynamic stabilizers.

Managing Scapular Dyskinesis 427

W. Ben Kibler, John William Lockhart, Robin Cromwell, and Aaron Sciascia

Scapular dyskinesis, the impairment of optimal scapular position and motion, is common in association with shoulder injury. A comprehensive evaluation process can show the causative factors and lead to effective treatment protocols. The complexity of scapular motion and the integrated relationship between the scapula, humerus, trunk, and legs suggest a need to develop rehabilitation programs that involve all segments working as a unit rather than isolated components. This is best accomplished with an integrated rehabilitation approach that includes rectifying deficits in mobility, strength, and motor control but not overtly focusing on any one area.

Adhesive Capsulitis 453

Nels Leafblad, Josh Mizels, Robert Tashjian, and Peter Chalmers

Adhesive capsulitis, colloquially known as "frozen shoulder," is a relatively common disorder, affecting approximately 2% to 5% of the general population. The incidence may be higher as the condition can be relatively mild and self-limited and thus many patients who experience it may never present for treatment. It involves a pathologic process of gradual fibrosis of the glenohumeral joint that leads to limited active and passive range of motion, contracture of the joint capsule, and shoulder pain.

Postoperative Rehabilitation After Shoulder Arthroplasty 469

William Polio and Tyler J. Brolin

Total shoulder arthroplasty (TSA), including anatomic TSA (aTSA) and reverse TSA (rTSA), has increased in popularity due to reliably good patient outcomes. Postoperative physical therapy (PT) is considered essential to the success of this operation and has become standard practice. The authors present general rehabilitation principles as well as preferred postoperative PT protocols for aTSA and rTSA, which are based on evidence-based literature and the different early postoperative concerns for each of these procedures.

Muscular Retraining and Rehabilitation after Shoulder Muscle Tendon Transfer 481

Abdulaziz F. Ahmed, Ryan Lohre, and Bassem T. Elhassan

Muscle tendon transfers around the shoulder involve transferring the tendon of a well-functioning muscle–tendon unit to the site of damaged muscle–tendon insertion. In turn, this restores function and strength of the injured shoulder muscle through dynamic muscular contraction and a tenodesis effect. Rehabilitation after shoulder muscle tendon transfers requires extensive and lengthy rehabilitation to achieve satisfactory clinical outcomes. It is crucial to gain detailed understanding of the rehabilitation requirements for different tendon transfer procedures such as the type of immobilization and specific range of motion limitations at specific time points during rehabilitations.

Brandon J. Erickson, Yousef Shishani, and Reuben Gobezie

Postoperative rehabilitation is a critical part of the treatment algorithm for patients with shoulder issues. When patients could not go to in-person therapy, many therapists pivoted to a remote option, and several application-based rehabilitation programs emerged. This article will discuss the shift to remote patient rehabilitation and will highlight the benefits and potential pitfalls of remote rehabilitation. It will also discuss ways to monitor patients remotely as they are performing their postoperative rehabilitation exercises. Finally, it will discuss how these remote platforms can be used, and what the user experience is like for the patient and the surgeon.

PHYSICAL MEDICINE AND REHABILITATION CLINICS OF NORTH AMERICA

FORTHCOMING ISSUES

August 2023
Post-Covid Rehabilitation
Monica Verduzco-Gutierrez, *Editor*

November 2023
Disorders of Consciousness
Sunil Kothari and Bei Zhang, *Editors*

February 2024
Burn Rehabilitation
Karen Kowalske, *Editor*

RECENT ISSUES

February 2023
Orthobiologics
Michael Khadavi and Luga Podesta, *Editors*

November 2022
Wound and Skin Care
Xiaohua Zhou and Cassandra Renfro, *Editors*

August 2022
Functional Medicine
Elizabeth Bradley, *Editor*

SERIES OF RELATED INTEREST

Orthopedic Clinics
https://www.orthopedic.theclinics.com/
Neurologic Clinics
https://www.neurologic.theclinics.com/
Clinics in Sports Medicine
https://www.sportsmed.theclinics.com/

VISIT THE CLINICS ONLINE!
Access your subscription at:
www.theclinics.com

PHYSICAL MEDICINE AND REHABILITATION CLINICS OF NORTH AMERICA

Foreword

A Fresh Review of Common Shoulder Conditions

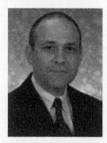

Santos F. Martinez, MD, MS
Consulting Editor

This issue of our musculoskeletal module focuses on common conditions involving the shoulder and takes us through the nonsurgical phases on through and including postsurgical treatment.

I have always had a very high regard for those practitioners whose chosen mission is dedicated to optimizing functional use of the upper extremity whether that be for use in the arts, sports, vocation, or for accomplishing the most basic activities of daily living. The shoulder girdle considerations are complex and cannot rest with confining one to a single joint. These encompass a combination of joints, whether they be true or functional joints, an unusual floating sesamoid (scapula), and array of musculoligamentous primary and secondary contributors. The synchronous contributors of this orchestra, which are composed of stabilizers and dynamic factors, with the input of inherent neural conductors contribute to a common objective. A journey more centrally takes us to axial contributors and connections, which project and facilitate motion from the lower extremities and trunk for accomplishing certain missions and demands of the upper extremity.

I am very honored to welcome Dr Throckmorton and his Orthopedic Surgical guests to share their knowledge for this collaborative effort. Dr Throckmorton has made such an impact as both an educator and a surgeon serving as a mentor for countless medical students, residents, and fellows at Campbell Clinic, which has been providing Orthopedic care for pediatric and adult populations for over a century.

I would also like to acknowledge two late exceptional educators. The first is in remembrance of Dr Carson D. Schneck, who dedicated greater than 50 years as an exemplary Anatomist/Physician at the Lewis Katz School of Medicine at Temple University in Philadelphia. His enthusiasm and detailed teaching were a major catalyst for students and surgeons alike. The second is Dr Alberto Inclan Costa, who was a

Phys Med Rehabil Clin N Am 34 (2023) xiii–xiv
https://doi.org/10.1016/j.pmr.2023.02.001
1047-9651/23/© 2023 Published by Elsevier Inc.

pioneer and orthopedic trailblazer in Latin America and founder of the Cuban Society of Orthopaedics and Traumatology.

Santos F. Martinez, MD, MS
Campbell Clinic
Department of Orthopaedic Surgery and
Biomedical Engineering
University of Tennessee College of Medicine
Memphis, TN 38104, USA

E-mail address:
smartinez@campbellclinic.com

Preface

Rehabilitation of Operative and Nonoperative Shoulder Pathologies

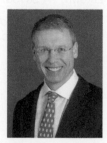

Thomas (Quin) Throckmorton, MD
Editor

On behalf of the authors of this issue of *Physical Medicine and Rehabilitation Clinics of North America*, we are pleased to present this issue entitled "Rehabilitation of Operative and Nonoperative Shoulder Pathologies". The articles herein are authored by experienced shoulder surgeons and thought-leaders in our field of orthopedic surgery. We hope that this issue will assist PM&R specialists in their treatment of patients with these disorders.

Rehabilitation of the shoulder, particularly following surgery, has been notoriously difficult to define and study. Due to the individualized nature of surgical recovery and differing philosophies among surgeons regarding the aggressiveness of physical therapy programs, high-level studies of shoulder rehabilitation have generally been lacking. Therefore, understanding in this area is often limited to institutional protocols. These authors have shared their extensive clinical experience in their particular areas of expertise to provide principles to guide rehabilitation after shoulder surgery.

Nonoperative shoulder pathologic conditions lend themselves better to more robust study, with rehabilitation protocols that are often well-defined and well-studied. These articles reflect this difference with analysis and discussion of high-level studies that can help guide practitioners in their treatment of these pathologic conditions. We hope that readers will gain valuable insight and understanding into shoulder rehabilitation protocols that can be used to benefit their patients.

On a personal level, I am very grateful to my friend and practice partner, Sandy Martinez, MD, who approached me about editing this issue. It has been a pleasure working with everyone involved to put this issue together. I would also like to dedicate this issue to my close friend and residency classmate, Clint Devin, MD, a renowned and highly published orthopedic spine surgeon who tragically was killed in a plane

Phys Med Rehabil Clin N Am 34 (2023) xv–xvi
https://doi.org/10.1016/j.pmr.2023.02.002
1047-9651/23/© 2023 Published by Elsevier Inc.

pmr.theclinics.com

crash in 2021. Clint was a pioneer in spine outcomes research, and I hope Clint would approve of the evidence-based recommendations we present here…even if they are from shoulder doctors.

Thomas (Quin) Throckmorton, MD
Shoulder and Elbow Surgery
University of Tennessee–Campbell Clinic
Department of Orthopaedic Surgery
1400 South Germantown Road
Germantown, TN 38138, USA

E-mail address:
tthrockmorton@campbellclinic.com

Shoulder Impingement Syndrome

Evan H. Horowitz, MD[a], William R. Aibinder, MD[b],*

KEYWORDS

- Shoulder • Impingement • Subacromial • Acromion • Subcoracoid • Rotator cuff
- Bursitis

KEY POINTS

- Shoulder pain has been cited as the third most common musculoskeletal pain complaint, with impingement syndrome as the most common diagnosis.
- The mainstay of treatment of shoulder impingement syndrome is nonoperative treatment.
- Refractory cases, or those with an objective or mechanical explanation for symptoms, may benefit from surgical intervention.

INTRODUCTION/BACKGROUND/PREVALENCE

Shoulder pain has been cited as the third most common musculoskeletal pain complaint with a prevalence between 7% and 30%.[1–5] Impingement syndrome is the most common diagnosis when evaluating shoulder pain.[6] This concept was first theorized by Neer in 1972, referring to impingement of the tendinous rotator cuff by the coracoacromial (CA) ligament and the anterior aspect of the acromion, with occasional involvement of bone spurring and osteophyte formation.[7] Recently, the term "shoulder impingement syndrome" has been questioned, highlighting the simplicity and broadness of the diagnosis, which may affect the ability of physicians and therapists to communicate effectively.[8–10] Thus, the purpose of this review will be to describe the anatomic basis of subacromial impingement, internal shoulder impingement, and subcoracoid impingement. We will focus primarily on the evaluation and diagnosis, as well as common nonsurgical treatment modalities. Surgical intervention is reserved for patients who fail conservative measures.

[a] Department of Orthopaedic Surgery and Rehabilitation Medicine, SUNY Downstate Health Sciences University, 450 Clarkson Avenue, MSC 30, Brooklyn, NY 11203, USA; [b] Department of Orthopaedic Surgery, University of Michigan, 24 Frank Lloyd Wright Drive, Ann Arbor, MI 48106, USA
* Corresponding author.
E-mail address: Waibinde@med.umich.edu
Twitter: @EvanHorowitzMD (E.H.H.); @WillAibinderMD (W.R.A.)

Phys Med Rehabil Clin N Am 34 (2023) 311–334
https://doi.org/10.1016/j.pmr.2022.12.001

SUBACROMIAL IMPINGEMENT

Subacromial impingement is thought to be due to both extrinsic and intrinsic theories.[11,12] Some authors support one theory over the other; however, it is likely a combination of both factors that leads to the pathology. Extrinsic compression of the rotator cuff occurs due to limited space between the humeral head and the anterior acromion, CA ligaments, and acromioclavicular (AC) joint. Some have suggested that tension on the CA ligament during abduction causes acromial ossification and osteophyte formation at the ligament insertion site.[7,13] Other studies have shown that all planes of motion result in contact on the CA ligament resulting in proliferation of acromial spurs.[14] Acromial shape and morphology also play a role in extrinsic compression and is discussed later in this section. It has been shown that while acromial morphology does not change with age, increased age does lead to more proliferative acromial spur formation.[15]

In addition to extrinsic compression, it is hypothesized that intrinsic degradation of the rotator cuff through diminished vascular supply, tensile forces on the rotator cuff, and tendon aging lead to the constellation of symptoms related to subacromial impingement.[11,16–19] Advocates of the intrinsic theory propose that damage to the supraspinatus tendon initiates a cascade of events that leads to subacromial impingement.[11] Tendon impairment leads to eccentric tension overload of the rotator cuff, glenohumeral instability, and superior humeral head migration, which in turn creates the extrinsic contact that leads to spurring and perpetuates subacromial impingement.[11,20]

PATIENT EVALUATION OVERVIEW—SUBACROMIAL IMPINGEMENT

Initial patient evaluation begins with a thorough subjective history, review of systems, physical examination, and relevant imaging. A careful subjective history of symptoms should focus on the duration of symptoms, mechanism of onset (traumatic vs atraumatic), aggravating and alleviating factors, character and severity of pain, location of pain, patient's activity level and goals, and treatment modalities that have been attempted, including physical or occupational therapy, orthotics/braces, creams/gels/ointments, medications, injections, and surgical procedures. For cases of subacromial, internal, and subcoracoid impingement, the history often contains an insidious and atraumatic onset of symptoms, pain in certain positions and at night, often without overt complaints of weakness. Once a thorough history is obtained, a complete shoulder examination should be performed with the focus to rule out any obvious signs of glenohumeral instability, full thickness rotator cuff tears, arthritic changes, scapular dyskinesia, or other structural causes of symptoms. Additionally, many of these may be present in the setting of impingement.

Physical Examination—Subacromial Impingement

A complete shoulder physical examination should be performed. The examination starts with inspections of the shoulder, and it is imperative to appropriately visualize the entire shoulder girdle in order to first inspect the shoulder. This includes the "6 S's": skin, scars, swelling, size, symmetry, and scapula.

Skin: Skin examination will often be normal in isolated shoulder impingement cases; however, areas of hypopigmentation may be related to prior corticosteroid injection sites.
Scars: Prior surgical scars may be present. The location, size, and number of scars may give clues about prior procedures. However, without imaging or prior operative reports, such information must be used cautiously because it is not objective.

Swelling: Assess for swelling that may be a sign of acute injury, which is nonspecific and may be from either trauma, overuse, or tearing of muscles, tendons, intra-articular, or ligamentous structures.

Size: Assess for atrophy and hypertrophy of the rotator cuff musculature. Atrophy may be a sign of disuse, frailty, hyponutrition, or in some cases, chronic muscle or tendon tears. Unilateral atrophy should also raise suspicion for peripheral nerve compression.

Symmetry: Assess for symmetry of the shoulder girdle, particularly in cases of uni-lateral complaints.

Scapula: Assess for scapular symmetry, both at rest and with shoulder motion.[21] Scapular dyskinesia can be more common in athletes such as throwing athletes. Scapular dyskinesia has been found in as many as 68% of patients with rotator cuff abnormalities, 94% of patients with labral tears, and essentially 100% of pa-tients with glenohumeral instability.[22-26] It can also be the primary cause of a pa-tient's impingement and thus treatment, particularly physical therapy, should focus on the scapular dysfunction.

Next, careful palpation of the shoulder should be performed. Subacromial impinge-ment often leads to diffuse pain; however, patients may report maximal tenderness at the rotator cuff insertion site on the greater tuberosity.

Passive range of motion (PROM) and active range of motion (AROM) should be eval-uated. In all cases of shoulder impingement, extremes of motion are usually limited by pain at points of compression; however, PROM is typically normal.

A detailed examination of the rotator cuff should be performed as well to include an empty can test (**Fig. 1A**),[26] drop arm sign (**Fig. 1B**),[26] external rotation lag sign (**Fig. 1C**),[27] Hornblower's sign (**Fig. 1D**),[28] belly press (**Fig. 1E**),[27] bear hug test (**Fig. 1F**),[29] and lift off test (**Fig. 1G**).[30] Any concern for a full thickness rotator cuff tear with cross weakness in any plane, particularly with a positive lag sign should prompt obtaining advanced imaging.

A full distal neurologic examination should be performed and documented, including motor, sensory, and reflex testing. The authors recommend performing a Spurling's test in patients who report any periscapular and/or neck pain.[31] To do so, the patient's neck is extended and rotated to the affected side, the head is laterally bent to the affected side, and the examiner applies vertical compression to the top of the head. This is a positive test if it reproduces symptoms in the ipsilateral arm. This test is specific but has poor sensitivity.[31]

Provocative tests for impingement are extremely useful. Studies have shown excel-lent correlation between examination findings and MRI findings when evaluating supraspinatus tears.[32] Additional MRI studies proved that these tests cause true me-chanical impingement that can be appreciated on imaging. These studies have found that the Hawkins test produced more subacromial space narrowing and impingement than the Neer test.[33,34] An additional study showed that shoulders in the Neer position demonstrated contact between the rotator cuff and the medial acromion, whereas shoulders in the Hawkins position produced contact between the rotator cuff and the CA ligament.[35]

Provocative Impingement Tests—Subacromial Impingement

The Neer impingement sign helps to indicate rotator cuff or bursal impingement against the CA arch. It has been shown to have sensitivity 72% and specificity 60%.[36] False positives occur due to stiffness, arthritis, instability, or osseous lesions. To perform the maneuver, the examiner stabilizes the scapula, places the arm in the

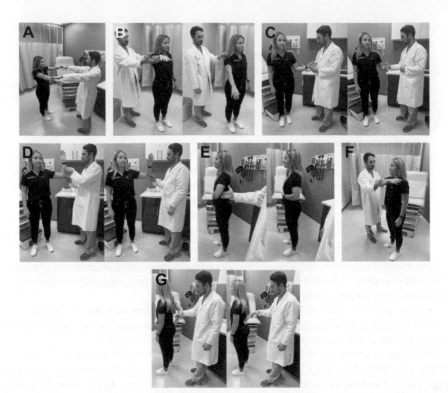

Fig. 1. Multiple examination tests have been described to evaluating the rotator cuff. Tests for the supraspinatus include the empty can (Jobe) test (*A*) and the drop arm sign (*B*). The Jobe test is performed by abducting the arm in the plane of the scapula, internally rotating the shoulder and having the patient resist a downward force, and the drop arm sign is performed by passively elevating the arm in the scapular plane to the horizontal and asking the patient to slowly drop the arm. Both tests are positive if painful or weak. Tests for external rotation include the external rotation lag sign (*C*) and the Hornblower's sign (*D*). The external rotation lag sign is performed by passively externally rotating the shoulder with the elbow flexed to 90° and then asking the patient hold while letting go. This tests the infraspinatus and is positive if the arm drifts into internal rotation. The Hornblower's sign is performed by abducting and externally rotating the shoulder to 90° and asking the patient hold this position while letting go. This tests the teres minor and is positive if the arm drifts into internal rotation. Tests for the subscapularis include the belly press test (*E*), the bear hug test (*F*), and the lift off test (*G*). The belly press test is performed by asking the patient to press the palm into the abdomen and bring the elbow forward to the plane of the body. This can also be performed as a lag sign as demonstrated in the picture. The test is positive if weakness and inability to maintain the elbow in front of the plane of the body. The bear hug test is performed by placing the hand on the contralateral arm and asking the patient to resist while applying an anterior force. The test is positive with weakness or pain. The lift off test is performed by placing the patient's hand with the palm posterior on the lower back and asking the patient to lift the arm posteriorly off the back. This can also be performed as a lag sign as demonstrated in the figure. The test is positive if weakness and inability to move or keep the hand off the back.

plane of the scapula, and the arm is passively raised. The test is positive if pain is elicited because the greater tuberosity impinges against the acromion (between 70° and 110°; **Fig. 2**).

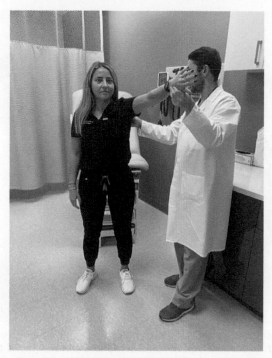

Fig. 2. Examiner performs the Neer impingement test with the right arm stabilizing the scapula while passively raising the arm.

The Neer impingement test is performed by repeating the impingement maneuver after injection of a local anesthetic into the subacromial space. If there is a decrease in pain, this is considered a positive sign.

The Hawkins test aims to cause impingement of the greater tuberosity underneath the CA ligament. It has been shown to have sensitivity of 79% and specificity of 59% for impingement.[36] To perform the maneuver, the examiner flexes the shoulder and elbow to 90°, and then internally rotates the arm. The test is considered positive if the symptoms of pain are recreated (**Fig. 3**).

Imaging Studies—Subacromial Impingement

Initial evaluation should begin with plain radiographs, which are typically normal in cases of impingement syndrome. The senior author's standard series includes a Grashey view, anteroposterior internal rotation view, scapular Y, and axillary lateral. In subacromial impingement, acromion morphology may play a role in the process. In 1986, Bigliani and colleagues classified acromion morphology.[37] They described 3 distinct types of acromial morphology; a fourth type (convex distal acromion) was later described by Vanarthos and colleagues in 1995.[38] Acromial morphology does not change with time but increased spurring occurs with age.[15] The types of acromia include a Type I (flat), Type II (curved), Type III (hooked), and Type IV (convex) (**Fig. 4**).[39]

The significance of acromial morphology in relation to impingement and rotator cuff tears is debated. Several authors reported that type III acromion is associated with shoulder impingement syndrome and rotator cuff tears.[40–42] However, other authors

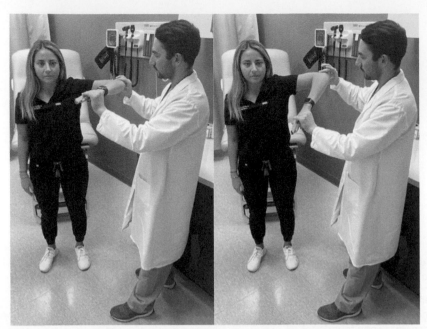

Fig. 3. Examiner performs the Hawkins test by passively applying an internal rotation force to the arm with 90° of forward flexion/abduction and the elbow flexed to 90°.

have contradicted these findings, and found instead that it is the acromial spurring that is associated with full-thickness rotator cuff tears but not partial tears.[43]

The critical shoulder angle (CSA) is a novel angle measured from the inferior pole of the glenoid and the glenoid plane to the lateral edge of the acromion (**Fig. 5**). In 2013, Moor and colleagues hypothesized that a smaller CSA would correlate with shoulder arthritis, and a larger CSA would correlate with rotator cuff tears.[44] They stated that the normal CSA range was between 30° and 35°.[44] Passaplan and colleagues in 2021 reported that the CSA measurement remains constant in patients and does not change over time.[45] Acceptance of the CSA as a predictor of rotator cuff tears has been inconsistent and its role in impingement syndrome has not been elucidated.[43,46–49]

Additional radiographic parameters for shoulder impingement syndrome diagnosis have been proposed. Amit and colleagues investigated the sharpened lateral acromion morphology (SLAM sign) (**Fig. 6**).[41] They measured the angle between the inferior and lateral borders of the acromion using the most inferolateral point as the apex and

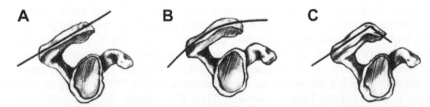

Fig. 4. The Bigliani Classification of acromial morphology, demonstrating a Type I or flat acromion (*A*), a Type II or curved acromion (*B*), and a Type III or hooked acromion (*C*). (*From* Bright, A., Torpey, B., Magid, D. et al. Reliability of radiographic evaluation for acromial morphology. Skeletal Radiol 26, 718–721 (1997).)

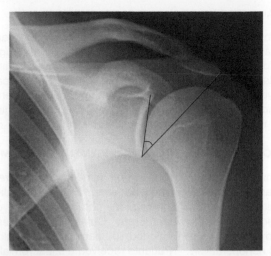

Fig. 5. Example of the CSA measured as the angle of the glenoid plane from the inferior pole of the glenoid to the lateral edge of the acromion.

termed this the "inferolateral acromion angle" (ILAA). If less than 90°, it was considered an SLAM sign. They compared this finding with acromial type III and the CSA greater than 35°. They found that all 3 imaging findings (acromial type, CSA, and SLAM sign) correlated to rotator cuff tears but the SLAM sign had the strongest correlation.[41]

Ultrasound is a useful and inexpensive imaging modality that has been shown to be accurate for full thickness rotator cuff tears, and bursitis of the subacromial or subdeltoid bursae. Early tendinitis changes are seen with high echogenicity and thickening. Bursitis is seen as a thickened bursa wall and anechoic effusion.[50–52] Thus, ultrasound may have some utility in the clinical setting with a well-trained operator.

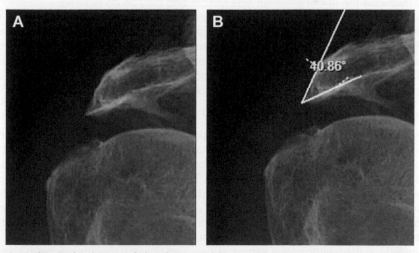

Fig. 6. Radiographic image of the sharpened lateral acromion morphology (*A*), with the ILAA measured at 40° (*B*), consistent with an SLAM sign. (*From* Amit P, Paluch AJ, Baring T. Sharpened lateral acromion morphology (SLAM sign) as an indicator of rotator cuff tear: a retrospective matched study. JSES Int. 2021 Jul 14;5(5):850-855. https://doi.org/10. 1016/j.jseint.2021.05.013. PMID: 34505095; PMCID: PMC8411071.)

CLASSIFICATION AND STAGING OF SUBACROMIAL IMPINGEMENT

Neer classified subacromial impingement into 3 stages.[53] Although rarely discussed in current clinical practices, the stages can help guide treatment. Stage 1 (edema and hemorrhage) is typically seen in patients aged younger than 25 years and managed conservatively. Stage II (fibrosis and tendinitis) is typically seen in patients aged between 25 and 40 years, which may require bursectomy or CA ligament division. Stage III (bone spurs and tendon rupture) is typically seen in patients aged older than 40 years, which may require anterior acromioplasty and/or rotator cuff repair.

TREATMENT OPTIONS FOR SUBACROMIAL IMPINGEMENT SYNDROME

Nonoperative management of subacromial impingement syndrome remains the mainstay of treatment and is successful in most patients.[54,55] Initial modalities include non-opioid pain medication such as nonsteroidal anti-inflammatory drugs (NSAIDs), corticosteroid injections, and physical therapy. Cummins and colleagues produced a prospective study, in 2009, which included 100 patients with shoulder impingement syndrome treated nonoperatively.[55] Patients received a subacromial cortisone injection and physical therapy. 79% of patients avoided surgery at 2-year follow-up. ASES scores increased from 56 to 95, and visual analog scale pain score decreased from 4.8 to 0.6. Total number of injections and patient response to the initial injection were predictors of future surgical interventions. Overall, their findings demonstrate that nonoperative management yields good outcomes.

Pharmacologic or medical treatment options

Several over the counter and prescription NSAIDs are commonly available. Given the longer half-life, the senior author prefers naproxen due to decreased dosing frequency.[56] Some NSAIDs have increased COX-2 selectivity over COX-1, which may lead to decreased gastrointestinal side effects; however, these medications have an increased risk of cardiovascular and clotting side effects.[57,58–60] Topical NSAIDs may decrease the risk of systemic side effects and may be considered.

Acetaminophen may be safer for use in patients with renal disease but should be avoided in patients with hepatic disease. It may provide symptom control in select patients but it does not decrease inflammation in the peripheral tissues. It inhibits the prostaglandin pathway within the central nervous system.[61] Although some patients and providers prefer acetaminophen for its lack of gastrointestinal and blood thinning side effect profile, it is not an anti-inflammatory medication.

Nonpharmacologic or surgical/interventional treatment options

Physical therapy including a home exercise program is very effective. In a systematic review, Kuhn demonstrated that exercise improves pain symptoms and function but not range of motion or strength.[60] Steuri and colleagues showed that guided exercises lead to better results than generic exercises.[62] Thus, patients should be started on a supervised therapy program, and they can advance to home exercises once they can demonstrate the exercises on their own and are showing improvement. Patients who do not require manual therapy techniques, and who have developed proficiency in the protocol may progress to an unsupervised home exercise program.[63]

Similarly, in the postoperative setting, supervised physical therapy has been shown to be superior to unsupervised home exercise programs following arthroscopic acromioplasty for impingement syndrome.[64]

Yet, studies have shown that manual therapy in addition to isolated physical therapy improves outcomes in patients with shoulder impingement syndrome.[65] Some reports note improvement in strength and function and decreased pain. Manual therapy techniques included soft tissue massage and muscle stretching focusing on the pectoralis minor, infraspinatus, teres minor, upper trapezius, sternocleidomastoid, and scalenes.[66,67]

Kuhn also described a thorough, evidence-based rehabilitation protocol for the treatment of rotator cuff impingement.[63] A summary of his 5 distinct categories is presented here and is the preferred guidelines for the senior author:

1. Modalities: Heat or cold, or both, may be used. The literature does not support the use of ultrasound treatment because results were similar between test subjects and controls.
2. Manual therapy: Joint and soft tissue mobilization techniques are useful during a period of supervised exercise. Patients should be instructed on a home exercise program and once able, should transition to one.
3. Range of motion: Begin with postural exercises such as shrugs and shoulder retraction to stabilize the scapula. Glenohumeral motion should be initiated with pendulum exercises. This can be progressed to active assisted motion and then active motion as tolerated. Active assisted motion can be performed by the patient using a cane, pulleys, or the uninvolved arm.
4. Flexibility: Daily stretching should be performed, for both the anterior and posterior shoulder. Stretches should be held for 30 seconds and repeated 5 times, with a 10-second rest in between stretches.
5. Strengthening: The focus of strengthening is the rotator cuff and scapular stabilizing muscles. Rotator cuff strengthening should be focused on internal rotation with the arm adducted at the side, external rotation with the arm adducted at the side, and scaption exercises if there is no associated pain. Scapular stabilization exercises include chair presses, push-ups, and upright rows. Standing forward elevation and extension exercises can be performed with elastic bands. Each exercise should be performed as 3 sets of 10 repetitions and may increase with patient progression.

Corticosteroid injections into the shoulder capitalize on the anti-inflammatory effects of steroids, which have been used in treating degenerative joint disease in other joints in the body. Steuri and colleagues demonstrated that corticosteroid injections were superior to placebo in the treatment of shoulder impingement syndrome.[62] Cuomo and colleagues performed a prospective, double-blinded, randomized control trial comparing steroid injections with plain lidocaine injections and found that 84% of steroid injection patients reported significant improvement in pain, and only 36% of controls reported improvement.[68] Additionally, 76% of the steroid group had improvement in activities of daily living (ADLs), whereas this was seen in only 23% of the lidocaine group.[68] Dong and colleagues reported that corticosteroid injections should be used in conjunction with therapy for best results, and worse effects are noted when corticosteroid injections are performed alone.[69] Patients should be counseled on the risks of corticosteroid injections before administration. Diabetic patients should be counseled to monitor their glucose levels. A hemoglobin A1c greater than 7% has been postulated as a cutoff for higher risk of postinjection day 1 increases in glucose.[70] All patients should be counseled on the risk of tendon rupture, which although rare, has been described.[71] Patients should be counseled on the risk of the "flare phenomenon," which is a paradoxic, short-term increase in pain following a corticosteroid injection, which is self-limiting in nature.[72] It should be discussed with the patient that shoulder surgery should be delayed after corticosteroid injection because risks of repair failure and postoperative infection may be increased.[73] Some authors advocate for a 6-month delay before performing shoulder tendon repair procedures following a local injection, although recent data may suggest that a shorter period is acceptable.[73] The risks of shoulder joint infection and local skin hypopigmentation should be discussed as well.

Hyaluronic acid is a long polysaccharide (glycosaminoglycan) chain with hydrophilicity, providing viscoelastic properties. It is theorized to provide mechanical properties similar to cartilage in the form of impact absorption, and synovial fluid in the form of joint lubrication.[74] Although hyaluronic acid injections have been studied and shown to demonstrate some success in the treatment of knee osteoarthritis, evidence is currently lacking in terms of replicating this success in the shoulder.[75] Penning and colleagues performed a randomized control trial, which demonstrated that hyaluronic acid injections for subacromial impingement syndrome did not provide improved results when compared with corticosteroid injections or placebo.[76] Hsieh redemonstrated this in a 2021 randomized control trial, showing that corticosteroid injections performed superior to hyaluronic acid injections; furthermore, they showed hyaluronic acid injections to be only marginally better than normal saline placebo injection.[77]

Additional Modalities

Additional modalities that have been proposed in the treatment of shoulder impingement syndrome include ultrasound, laser therapy, pulsed electromagnetic field treatment, extracorporeal shockwave therapy (ECSWT), taping, and hyperthermia. Definitive evidence to support these is lacking. In a randomized control trial, Shakeri and colleagues demonstrated that kinesiological taping was able to demonstrate significant decreases in motion-related pain and nocturnal pain when compared with placebo taping,[78] and other authors demonstrated that taping may be effective in the early stages of shoulder impingement syndrome.[69] Steuri and colleagues used meta-analysis to compile low-quality evidence reporting that laser treatment, ECSWT, and taping may be superior to sham treatment.[62] An analysis of 2 systematic reviews and 10 randomized control trials evaluated the use of exercise therapy, ultrasound, laser, pulsed electromagnetic field, and hyperthermia for subacromial impingement syndrome.[79] Moderate evidence supported hyperthermia and exercise therapy in the short term; however, lasting effects were unable to be shown for any intervention aside from exercise therapy.

Surgical Options and Outcomes—Subacromial Impingement Syndrome

Surgical intervention is reserved for patients who fail a trial of nonoperative treatment measures. The mainstay of operative intervention is open or arthroscopic subacromial decompression, which includes an acromioplasty with CA ligament release. In 1972, Neer introduced the idea of anterior acromioplasty with release of the CA ligament in the treatment of subacromial impingement.[7] Although his originally described procedure was open and not arthroscopic, the study reported good results in terms of pain relief in patients with chronic pain from subacromial impingement. The principles of anterior acromioplasty include removing the anterior edge and undersurface of the anterior acromion, the attached CA ligament, biceps tendon decompression and removal of groove osteophytes, and resection of hypertrophic spurring at the AC joint.[7]

Ellman described the arthroscopic subacromial decompression technique in 1987.[80] About 88% of patients had a satisfactory result with 88% also returning to their prior level of sporting activity. A 2010 meta-analysis showed equivalent outcomes, operative times, and complication rates between open and arthroscopic methods.[81] Additional studies have shown good results regarding pain relief in these patients.[11,82]

Potential complications include deltoid dysfunction and anterosuperior escape. Care should be taken to not resect an excessive amount of anterior acromion near the deltoid attachment. Preoperative imaging should be inspected for os acromiale because complete excision can cause deltoid dysfunction. Anterosuperior escape can occur if acromioplasty and CA ligament release are performed in patients with massive rotator cuff tears.

In a cadaveric study, Colman and colleagues found that flattening of the anterior ridge removed an average thickness of 1.9 + 0.5 mm of bone and only removed impingement in 50% of specimens, whereas flattening of the anterior third to the midline removed an average of 5.4 + 1.9 mm of bone and eliminated impingement in 100% of cases.[83] No further benefit was gained by the most aggressive resection or flattening of the entire acromion.

INTERNAL IMPINGEMENT

Internal impingement, in contrast, is primarily an intra-articular pathologic condition that is characterized by excessive or repetitive impact of the greater tuberosity with the posterosuperior glenoid. This occurs with arm abduction and external rotation (ABER), the so-called late cocking phase of throwing.[84] Internal impingement results in articular-sided rotator cuff degeneration and posterior labral tears or fraying (**Fig. 7**). The pathoanatomy is thought to be multifactorial and includes glenohumeral instability, scapular dyskinesis, and posterior shoulder capsule tightness. Common findings include posterior glenohumeral joint line tenderness, decreased internal rotation, increased external rotation, and pain in the abducted and external rotation position.

PATIENT EVALUATION OVERVIEW—INTERNAL IMPINGEMENT

Initial patient evaluation for internal impingement is similar to that of subacromial impingement and should begin with a thorough subjective history, review of systems, physical examination, and relevant imaging. This is detailed in the subacromial impingement section.

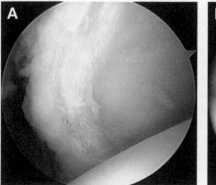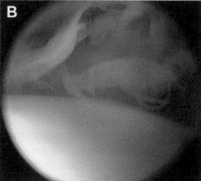

Fig. 7. Intraoperative arthroscopic view of the (A) posterior labrum fraying and the (B) articular side of the infraspinatus demonstrating fraying and degeneration in a patient with internal impingement. These are original images from the senior author.

Physical examination—internal impingement

In the evaluation of internal impingement, a complete shoulder physical examination should be performed. The overall physical examination is similar to that of subacromial impingement. The "6 S's" as outlined above should be performed: skin, scars, swelling, size, symmetry, and scapula. PROM and AROM should be evaluated and may demonstrate pain at the extreme of ABER. A full distal neurologic examination and rotator cuff examination should be performed and documented and previously outlined.

Next, careful palpation of the shoulder should be performed. Posterior glenohumeral joint line tenderness is suggestive of internal impingement, most likely at the posterosuperior glenoid and labrum.[84]

Provocative impingement tests for internal impingement

Provocative tests for impingement are extremely useful and include the internal impingement/posterior impingement sign and the relocation sign. Meister and colleagues studied the posterior impingement sign to attempt to reproduce posteriorly located pain.[85] The goal of the test is to cause impingement of the articular-sided rotator cuff and labrum between the glenoid and the greater tuberosity. Sensitivity was shown to be 75.5% and specificity was 85% for internal impingement.[85] When only noncontact athletes with posterior shoulder pain were included, sensitivity improved to 95% and specificity to 100%. Positive findings highly correlated with undersurface rotator cuff or posterior labrum tearing during arthroscopy, which were amenable to treatment. To perform this maneuver, the arm is placed in 90° to 110° of abduction and maximally externally rotated to recreate the late cocking phase. The arm is then extended 10° to 15°, and pain in this position is considered a positive test. External rotation in forward flexion rather than abduction should resolve the pain (**Fig. 8**).

The relocation sign was described by Jobe and colleagues with the arm abducted to 90° and maximally externally rotated (**Fig. 9**).[84,86,87] Pain in this position and resolution of pain with a posteriorly directed force on the proximal humerus is considered a positive test. During arthroscopic examination in 41 professional overhand throwing athletes with a positive test, the authors found 100% had either rotator cuff/posterosuperior glenoid contact, or osteochondral lesions.[88]

Imaging studies—internal impingement

Similar to subacromial impingement, in the evaluation of internal impingement, the initial evaluation should begin with plain radiographs. On plain film radiographs, some radiographic findings may be seen with internal impingement to assist with the diagnosis.[84] These include exostosis of the posteroinferior glenoid rim (Bennett lesion), sclerosis of the greater tuberosity, posterior humeral head osteochondral lesions or cysts, and rounding of the posterior glenoid rim.[84,89]

However, in the evaluation of internal impingement syndrome, MRI plays a larger role. Studies have evaluated MRI in shoulders with arthroscopically diagnosed internal impingement syndrome and have defined 3 distinct findings that are consistent with the diagnosis: (1) undersurface tears of the supraspinatus or infraspinatus, (2) cystic changes in the posterior aspect of the humeral head, and (3) posterior superior labral pathologic condition (**Fig. 10**).[90]

Fessa and colleagues proposed that shoulder positioning plays an important role during MRI when evaluating internal impingement.[91] The authors proposed that the shoulder position of ABER, which allows the posterosuperior rotator cuff to relax and allows

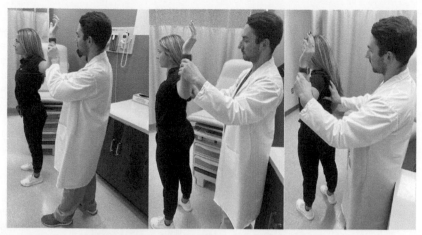

Fig. 8. Examiner performs the posterior impingement test by placing the arm in 90° to 110° of abduction and maximally externally rotated to recreate the late cocking phase. The arm is then extended 10° to 15° and pain in this position is considered a positive test.

more contrast into the tear. This position also places the humeral head and glenoid impaction sites closer together, and approximates the potential pathologic sites.

Treatment Options for Internal Impingement Syndrome

Similar to subacromial impingement, nonoperative management remains the mainstay of treatment. Initial modalities include nonopioid pain medication, corticosteroid injections, and physical therapy. Additional modalities that have been proposed in the treatment of shoulder impingement syndrome include ultrasound, laser therapy, pulsed electromagnetic field treatment, ECSWT, taping, and hyperthermia. These interventions are outlined in detail above, with inconclusive data.

For internal impingement, an intra-articular injection is preferred, and the authors' preferred technique is a posterior injection site located approximately 2 cm distal and medial to the posterolateral edge of the acromion. The injection can yield both therapeutic and diagnostic benefit.

Surgical options and outcomes—internal impingement

Internal impingement is associated with a high rate of concomitant pathologic condition, including biceps tenosynovitis, labral tears, and arthritic changes.[92] ElAttrache and colleagues demonstrated concomitant pathologic condition arthroscopically in overhand throwing athletes, finding that 93% of internal impingement patients had undersurface rotator cuff fraying, and 88% had posterosuperior labral fraying.[88] Treatment of this concomitant pathologic condition should be addressed based on the severity of the individual pathologic condition. For example, the amount of rotator cuff tearing to warrant debridement versus repair is a topic of debate. In 1985, Andrews and colleagues published on 36 overhead athletes who underwent debridement for articular-sided partial tears and demonstrated that 85% returned to premorbid function.[93] To further complicate the picture, it is possible that microinstability in the glenohumeral joint contributes to internal impingement pathologic condition, which, if unaddressed, can lead to continued pain, as theorized by Levitz and colleagues[94] Some have proposed the importance of addressing osseous pathologic condition such as the Bennett lesion or even performing a humeral osteotomy to change humeral version in refractory cases that failed arthroscopic management.[95,96]

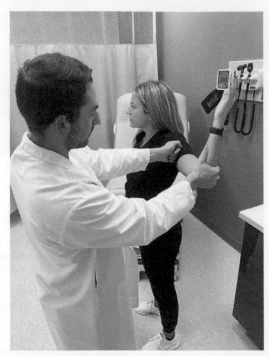

Fig. 9. Examiner performs the relocation sign by applying a posteriorly directed force on the proximal humerus, which should relieve pain.

Outcomes are difficult to study and vary based on the true intra-articular pathologic condition identified.

SUBCORACOID IMPINGEMENT

Subcoracoid impingement refers to pain due to compression of the subscapularis between the lesser tuberosity and the coracoid. Pain is usually located anteriorly and tearing of the subscapularis may occur.[97] Symptoms are reproduced with the arm adducted, forward flexed, and internally rotated. Coracoid morphology, such as a more lateral projection and shorter distance may predispose patients to this condition.[98] Some authors suggest that rotator cuff integrity and humeral head stability also play a role in this rare condition that requires a high index of suspicion.[99]

PATIENT EVALUATION OVERVIEW—SUBCORACOID IMPINGEMENT

Initial patient evaluation for internal impingement is similar to that of subacromial and internal impingement and should begin with a thorough subjective history, review of systems, physical examination, and relevant imaging.

Physical Examination—Subcoracoid Impingement

In the evaluation of subcoracoid impingement, a complete shoulder physical examination should be performed. The overall physical examination is similar to that of subacromial and internal impingement. The "6 S's" as outlined above should be performed: skin, scars, swelling, size, symmetry, and scapula. PROM and AROM should be

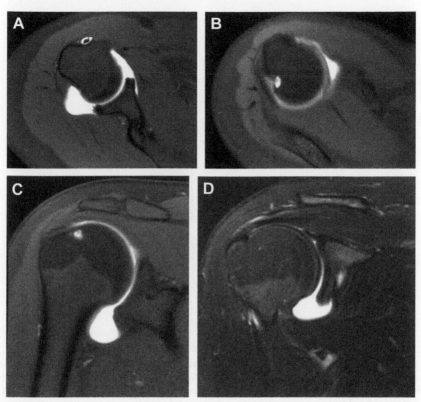

Fig. 10. MRI arthrogram of the patient in **Fig. 2,** which demonstrates (A) fraying of the posterior labrum on an axial slice, as well as (B, C) a posterosuperior osseous cyst seen on the axial and coronal slices, as well as (D) degenerative tearing of the posterosuperior rotator cuff tissue.

evaluated. A full distal neurovascular examination and rotator cuff examination should be performed and documented and previously outlined.

Next, careful palpation of the shoulder should be performed. Subcoracoid impingement patients may locate a single, focal point of tenderness anteriorly, at either the anterior coracoid or the lesser tuberosity.

Provocative Impingement Tests for Subcoracoid Impingement

Provocative tests for subcoracoid impingement are extremely useful and include pain induced by forward elevation and internal rotation of the arm. It is greatest between 120° and 130° of flexion. This is a higher degree of flexion than what is expected in subacromial impingement.

The coracoid impingement test is performed by placing the shoulder passively in a position of cross-arm adduction, forward elevation, and internal rotation to bring the lesser tuberosity in contact with the coracoid (**Fig. 11**). A positive test produces a painful clicking in the anterior shoulder.[100]

Imaging Studies—Subcoracoid Impingement

Similar to subacromial and internal impingement, in the evaluation of subcoracoid impingement, the initial evaluation should begin with plain radiographs.

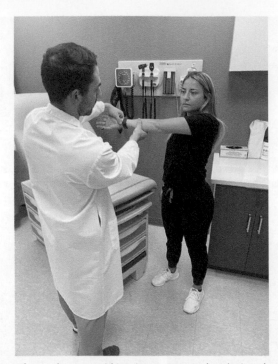

Fig. 11. Examiner performs the coracoid impingement test by placing the shoulder passively in a position of cross-arm adduction, forward elevation, and internal rotation to bring the lesser tuberosity in contact with the coracoid. A positive test produces a painful clicking in the anterior shoulder.

MRI and computed tomography (CT) play a significant role in the diagnosis of subcoracoid impingement. Some authors have used cine, or dynamic, MRI imaging, which allows use of a shoulder rotating device for a series of images in progressive rotating positions of the shoulder.[101] One study demonstrated that cine MRI can be a very useful tool in the diagnosis of subcoracoid impingement when other methods are inadequate (**Fig. 12**).[97]

CT scans are obtained with the arms crossed on the chest. A coracohumeral distance less than 6 mm is consistent with subcoracoid impingement. A normal distance is 8.7 mm with the arm adducted and 6.8 mm with the arm flexed.[98] Nonetheless, subcoracoid impingement is a clinical diagnosis, and a normal coracohumeral distance does not rule out the condition.[102]

TREATMENT OPTIONS FOR SUBCORACOID IMPINGEMENT SYNDROME

Similar to subacromial and internal impingement, nonoperative management is the mainstay of treatment and is similar to the other forms of impingement. In regard to injections, an ultrasound-guided injection is recommended to be performed by a trained specialist. Typically, this is performed with the arm at the side and external rotated to avoid subscapularis or biceps tendon involvement. Injection should be deep and lateral to the coracoid tip to maximize the therapeutic and diagnostic benefit.[97]

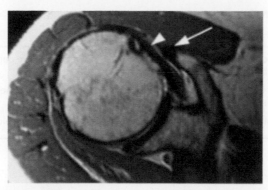

Fig. 12. Axial MRI image showing subcoracoid impingement. The arrowhead depicts the subscapularis with intrasubstance tendinosis, and the arrow demonstrates the elongated coracoid and decreased coracohumeral distance. (*From* Freehill, Michael Q. MD. Coracoid Impingement: Diagnosis and Treatment. American Academy of Orthopaedic Surgeon: April 2011 - Volume 19 - Issue 4 - p 191-197.)

Surgical options and outcomes—subcoracoid impingement

Surgical management is rare but may include arthroscopic coracoplasty with or without subscapularis tendon repair if indicated. The posterolateral coracoid should be resected to create a minimum of 7 mm of clearance between the coracoid and the subscapularis. Care should be taken to be aware of the dangers during arthroscopy for subcoracoid impingement, which include the musculocutaneous nerve, which is an average of 2.74 cm from the coracoid, the axillary nerve, which is an average of 3.5 cm from the coracoid, and the cephalic vein, which is an average of 1.37 cm from the coracoid.[103] Another option includes open coracoplasty, which includes resected the lateral portion of the coracoid. Then, the conjoined tendon is reattached to the remaining medial coracoid.[100] Reported surgical outcomes have been good and can be recommended for patients who have failed nonoperative measures.[100]

SUMMARY/DISCUSSION

Shoulder impingement syndrome has been cited as the most common cause of shoulder pain. The term "shoulder impingement syndrome" has been criticized as vague and nonspecific, and therefore misleading. Although shoulder impingement syndrome is likely multifactorial, the 3 most common subtypes would include subacromial impingement, internal impingement, and subcoracoid impingement. The mainstay of treatment is nonsurgical, as the majority of patients will improve with conservative measures. Surgical intervention is reserved for patients who fail conservative measures. Surgical intervention is most commonly in the form of decompression, with attention given to concomitant, associated pathologic condition of the shoulder, which commonly exists in the setting of impingement. The authors strongly emphasize that the specific subtype of shoulder impingement syndrome terminology be clearly communicated, as ambiguity can lead to misdiagnosis. Vague diagnoses such as "shoulder impingement syndrome" can lead to treatments that have a low likelihood of success because specific pathologic condition may go unaddressed.[104,105]

Finally, there is a clear need for future high-powered, high-quality, prospective randomized controlled trials in this arena in order to improve outcomes in patients with different impingement syndromes of the shoulder.

CLINICS CARE POINTS

- Supervised physical therapy and exercises have been shown to improve pain and function in the setting of subacromial impingement syndrome.
- In the sertting of internal impingement refractory to nonoperative treatment, articular sided debridement yields a reasonable return to function.
- A coracohumeral distance of less than 6 mm is consistent with subcoracoid impingement.

DISCLOSURE

E.H. Horowitz has nothing to disclose. W.R. Aibinder is a consultant for Exactech Inc, serves on the editorial board for EJOST.

REFERENCES

1. Urwin M, Symmons D, Allison T, et al. Estimating the burden of musculoskeletal disorders in the community: the comparative prevalence of symptoms at different anatomical sites, and the relation to social deprivation. Ann Rheum Dis 1998;57(11):649–55. PMID: 9924205; PMCID: PMC1752494.
2. Feleus A, Bierma-Zeinstra SM, Miedema HS, et al. Incidence of non-traumatic complaints of arm, neck and shoulder in general practice. Man Ther 2008; 13(5):426–33. Epub 2007 Aug 2. PMID: 17681866.
3. gutiérrez-Espinoza H, Araya-Quintanilla F, Cereceda-Muriel C, et al. Effect of supervised physiotherapy versus home exercise program in patients with subacromial impingement syndrome: A systematic review and meta-analysis. Phys Ther Sport 2020;41:34–42. Epub 2019 Nov 6. PMID: 31726386.
4. van der Windt DA, Koes BW, de Jong BA, et al. Shoulder disorders in general practice: incidence, patient characteristics, and management. Ann Rheum Dis 1995;54(12):959–64. PMID: 8546527; PMCID: PMC1010060.
5. Luime JJ, Koes BW, Hendriksen IJ, et al. Prevalence and incidence of shoulder pain in the general population; a systematic review. Scand J Rheumatol 2004; 33(2):73–81.
6. Michener LA, McClure PW, Karduna AR. Anatomical and biomechanical mechanisms of subacromial impingement syndrome. Clin Biomech (Bristol, Avon) 2003;18(5):369–79. PMID: 12763431.
7. Neer CS 2nd. Anterior acromioplasty for the chronic impingement syndrome in the shoulder: a preliminary report. J Bone Joint Surg Am 1972;54(1):41–50. PMID: 5054450.
8. Lewis J. The End of an Era? J Orthop Sports Phys Ther 2018;48(3):127–9.
9. Papadonikolakis, Anastasios MD1, McKenna Mark MD1, et al. MD1. Published Evidence Relevant to the Diagnosis of Impingement Syndrome of the Shoulder. J Bone Joint Surg 2011;93(19):1827–32.
10. Ludewig PM, Lawrence RL, Braman JP. What's in a Name? Using Movement System Diagnoses Versus Pathoanatomic Diagnoses. J Orthop Sports Phys Ther 2013;43(5):280–3.
11. Harrison AK, Flatow EL. Subacromial Impingement Syndrome. Am Acad Orthopaedic Surgeon 2011;19(11):701–8.
12. Lewis JS. Rotator cuff tendinopathy. Br J Sports Med 2009;43(4):236–41. Epub 2008 Sep 18. PMID: 18801774.

13. Chambler AF, Bull AM, Reilly P, et al. Coracoacromial ligament tension in vivo. J Shoulder Elbow Surg 2003;12(4):365–7. PMID: 12934032.
14. Yamamoto N, Muraki T, Sperling JW, et al. Contact between the coracoacromial arch and the rotator cuff tendons in nonpathologic situations: a cadaveric study. J Shoulder Elbow Surg 2010;19(5):681–7. Epub 2010 Mar 19. PMID: 20303292.
15. Nicholson GP, Goodman DA, Flatow EL, et al. The acromion: morphologic condition and age-related changes. A study of 420 scapulas. J Shoulder Elbow Surg 1996;5(1):1–11.
16. Lohr JF, Uhthoff HK. The microvascular pattern of the supraspinatus tendon. Clin Orthop Relat Res 1990;254:35–8. PMID: 2323147.
17. Chansky HA, Iannotti JP. The vascularity of the rotator cuff. Clin Sports Med 1991;10(4):807–22. PMID: 1934098.
18. Fukuda H, Hamada K, Yamanaka K. Pathology and pathogenesis of bursal-side rotator cuff tears viewed from en bloc histologic sections. Clin Orthop Relat Res 1990;254:75–80. PMID: 2323150.
19. Ogata S, Uhthoff HK. Acromial enthesopathy and rotator cuff tear. A radiologic and histologic postmortem investigation of the coracoacromial arch. Clin Orthop Relat Res 1990;254:39–48. PMID: 2323148.
20. Budoff JE, Nirschl RP, Guidi EJ. Debridement of partial-thickness tears of the rotator cuff without acromioplasty. Long-term follow-up and review of the literature. J Bone Joint Surg Am 1998;80(5):733–48. PMID: 9611036.
21. Martin RM, Fish DE. Scapular winging: anatomical review, diagnosis, and treatments. Curr Rev Musculoskelet Med 2008;1(1):1–11. PMID: 19468892; PMCID: PMC2684151.
22. Kibler WB, McMullen J. Scapular dyskinesis and its relation to shoulder pain. J Am Acad Orthop Surg 2003;11(2):142–51. PMID: 12670140.
23. Warner JJ, Micheli LJ, Arslanian LE, et al. Scapulothoracic motion in normal shoulders and shoulders with glenohumeral instability and impingement syndrome. A study using Moiré topographic analysis. Clin Orthop Relat Res 1992;285:191–9. PMID: 1446436.
24. Paletta GA Jr, Warner JJ, Warren RF, et al. Shoulder kinematics with two-plane x-ray evaluation in patients with anterior instability or rotator cuff tearing. J Shoulder Elbow Surg 1997;6(6):516–27. PMID: 9437601.
25. Burkhart SS, Morgan CD, Kibler WB. Shoulder injuries in overhead athletes. The "dead arm" revisited. Clin Sports Med 2000;19(1):125–58. PMID: 10652669.
26. Balevi B.E., Sarikaya P.Z.B., Kaygisiz, M.E., et al., Diagnostic dilemma: which clinical tests are most accurate for diagnosing supraspinatus muscle tears and tendinosis when compared to magnetic resonance imaging?, Cureus, 14 (6), 2022, e25903.
27. Schmidt M., Enger, M., Prill A.H., et al., Interrater reliability of physical examination tests in the acute phase of shoulder injuries, BMC Musculoskelet Disord, 22 (1), 2021, 770.
28. Walch G, Boulahia A, Calderone S, et al. The 'dropping' and 'Hornblower's' signs in evaluation of rotator-cuff tears. JBJS Br 1998;80(4):624–8.
29. Barth JRH, Burkhard SS, De Beer JF. The bear-hug test: a new and sensitive test for diagnosing a subscapularis tear. Arthroscopy 2006;22(10):1076–84.
30. Gerber C, Krushell RJ. Isolated rupture of the tendon of the subscapularis muscle. Clinical features in 16 cases. JBJS Br 1991;73(3):389–94.
31. Jones S.J. and John-Mark M.M., Spurling test, In: StatPearls, 2021, StatPearls Publishing: Treasure Island; FL.

32. Yazigi Junior JA, Anauate Nicolao F, Matsunaga FT, et al. Supraspinatus tears: predictability of magnetic resonance imaging findings based on clinical examination. J Shoulder Elbow Surg 2021;30(8):1834–43. Epub 2021 Mar 4. PMID: 33675978.

33. Pappas GP, Blemker SS, Beaulieu CF, et al. In vivo anatomy of the Neer and Hawkins sign positions for shoulder impingement. J Shoulder Elbow Surg 2006;15(1):40–9.

34. Roberts CS, Davila JN, Hushek SG, et al. Magnetic resonance imaging analysis of the subacromial space in the impingement sign positions. J Shoulder Elbow Surg 2002;11(6):595–9.

35. Valadie AL 3rd, Jobe CM, Pink MM, et al. Anatomy of provocative tests for impingement syndrome of the shoulder. J Shoulder Elbow Surg 2000;9(1): 36–46.

36. Hegedus E.J., Goode A.P., Cook C.E.,et al., Which physical examination tests provide clinicians with the most value when examining the shoulder? Update of a systematic review with meta-analysis of individual tests, Br J Sports Med, 46 (14), 2012, 964–978.

37. Bigliani LU, Morrison DS, April EW. The Morphology of the Acromion and Its Relationship to Rotator Cuff Tears. Orthopaedic Trans 1986;10:228.

38. Vanarthos WJ, Monu JU. Type 4 acromion: a new classification. Contemp Orthopaedics 1995;30(3):227–9. PMID: 10150316.

39. Bright AS, Torpey B, Magid T. Reliability of radiographic evaluation for acromial morphology. Skeletal Radiol 1997;26:718–21.

40. Epstein RE, Schweitzer ME, Frieman BG, et al. Hooked acromion: prevalence on MR images of painful shoulders. Radiology 1993;187(2):479–81.

41. Amit P, Paluch AJ, Baring T. Sharpened lateral acromion morphology (SLAM sign) as an indicator of rotator cuff tear: a retrospective matched study. JSES Int 2021;5(5):850–5. PMID: 34505095; PMCID: PMC8411071.

42. Toivonen DA, Tuite MJ, Orwin JF. Acromial structure and tears of the rotator cuff. J Shoulder Elbow Surg 1995;4(5):376–83.

43. Pandey V, Vijayan D, Tapashetti S, et al. Does scapular morphology affect the integrity of the rotator cuff? J Shoulder Elbow Surg 2016;25(3):413–21. Epub 2015 Dec 2. PMID: 26652696.

44. Moor BK, Bouaicha S, Rothenfluh DA, et al. Is there an association between the individual anatomy of the scapula and the development of rotator cuff tears or osteoarthritis of the glenohumeral joint?: A radiological study of the critical shoulder angle. Bone Joint J 2013;95-B(7):935–41.

45. Passaplan C, Hasler A, Gerber C. The critical shoulder angle does not change over time: a radiographic study. J Shoulder Elbow Surg 2021;30(8):1866–72. Epub 2020 Nov 4. PMID: 33160027.

46. Lin CL, Chen YW, Lin LF, et al. Accuracy of the Critical Shoulder Angle for Predicting Rotator Cuff Tears in Patients With Nontraumatic Shoulder Pain. Orthop J Sports Med 2020;8(5). 2325967120918995.

47. İncesoy MA, Yıldız KI, Türk Öİ, et al. The critical shoulder angle, the acromial index, the glenoid version angle and the acromial angulation are associated with rotator cuff tears. Knee Surg Sports Traumatol Arthrosc 2021;29(7):2257–63. Epub 2020 Jul 15. PMID: 32671437.

48. Kim JH, Min YK, Gwak HC, et al. Rotator cuff tear incidence association with critical shoulder angle and subacromial osteophytes. J Shoulder Elbow Surg 2019; 28(3):470–5. Epub 2018 Nov 12. PMID: 30429059.

49. Chalmers PN, Salazar D, Steger-May K, et al. Does the Critical Shoulder Angle Correlate With Rotator Cuff Tear Progression? Clin Orthop Relat Res 2017;475(6):1608–17. Epub 2017 Jan 24. PMID: 28120293; PMCID: PMC54 06338.

50. Daghir AA, Sookur PA, Shah S, et al. Dynamic ultrasound of the subacromial-subdeltoid bursa in patients with shoulder impingement: a comparison with normal volunteers. Skeletal Radiol 2012;41(9):1047–53. Epub 2011 Oct 14. PMID: 21997670.

51. Kloth JK, Zeifang F, Weber MA. Klinische oder radiologische Diagnose des Impingements [Clinical or radiological diagnosis of impingement]. Radiologe 2015;55(3):203–10. German.

52. Garving C, Jakob S, Bauer I, et al. Impingement syndrome of the shoulder. Dtsch Arztebl Int 2017;114:765–76.

53. Neer CS 2nd. Impingement lesions. Clin Orthop Relat Res 1983;173:70–7. PMID: 6825348.

54. Bigliani LU, Levine WN. Subacromial impingement syndrome. J Bone Joint Surg Am 1997;79(12):1854–68. PMID: 9409800.

55. Cummins CA, Sasso LM, Nicholson D. Impingement syndrome: temporal outcomes of nonoperative treatment. J Shoulder Elbow Surg 2009;18(2):172–7.

56. Elliot V.H. and Raymond A.D., Ch 17 - Nonopioid analgesics, In: Frank J.D., Angelo J.M., et al., Pharmacology and therapeutics for dentistry, 7th edition, 2017, Mosby: St. Louis, MO, 257–275, 9780323393072.

57. Smith H.S., Nonsteroidal anti-inflammatory drugs; acetaminophen, In: Michael J.A. and Robert B.D., Encyclopedia of the neurological sciences, 2nd edition, 2014, Academic Press: USA, 610–613, 9780123851581.

58. Hawkey C, Kahan A, Steinbrück K, et al. Gastrointestinal tolerability of meloxicam compared to diclofenac in osteoarthritis patients. International MELISSA Study Group. Meloxicam Large-scale International Study Safety Assessment. Br J Rheumatol 1998;37(9):937–45. Erratum in: Br J Rheumatol 1998;37(10): 1142. PMID: 9783757.

59. Stiller Carl-Olav, Paul Hjemdahl. Lessons from 20 years with COX-2 inhibitors: Importance of dose-response considerations and fair play in comparative trials. J Intern Med 2022;292(4):557–74.

60. Schmidt Morten, et al. Cardiovascular Risks of Diclofenac Versus Other Older COX-2 Inhibitors (Meloxicam and Etodolac) and Newer COX-2 Inhibitors (Celecoxib and Etoricoxib): A Series of Nationwide Emulated Trials. Drug Saf 2022; 45(9):983–94.

61. Graham GG, Scott KF. Mechanism of action of paracetamol. Am J Ther 2005; 12(1):46–55.

62. Steuri R, Sattelmayer M, Elsig S, et al. Effectiveness of conservative interventions including exercise, manual therapy and medical management in adults with shoulder impingement: a systematic review and meta-analysis of RCTs. Br J Sports Med 2017;51:1340–7.

63. Kuhn JE. Exercise in the treatment of rotator cuff impingement: a systematic review and a synthesized evidence-based rehabilitation protocol. J Shoulder Elbow Surg 2009;18(1):138–60.

64. Holmgren T, Oberg B, Sjöberg I, et al. Supervised strengthening exercises versus home-based movement exercises after arthroscopic acromioplasty: a randomized clinical trial. J Rehabil Med 2012;44(1):12–8.

65. Bang MD, Deyle GD. Comparison of supervised exercise with and without manual physical therapy for patients with shoulder impingement syndrome. J Orthop Sports Phys Ther 2000;30(3):126–37.

66. Hengeveld E, Banks K, Maitland GD. Maitland's peripheral manipulation. 5th edition. Edinburgh: Elsevier/Butterworth Heinemann; 2014. p. 142–260.

67. Olaf E& Jern H. Muscle Stretching in Manual Therapy: A Clinical Manual. Alfta Rehab. Volume I: The Extremities. 2002. ISBN 91-85934-02-X.

68. Cuom F, Blair B, et al. An Analysis of the Efficacy of Corticosteroid Injections for the Treatment of Subacromial Impingement Syndrome. J Shoulder Elbow Surg 1996;5(2):S8–9.

69. Dong W, Goost H, Lin XB, et al. Treatments for shoulder impingement syndrome: a PRISMA systematic review and network meta-analysis. Medicine (Baltimore) 2015;94(10):e510. Erratum in: Medicine (Baltimore). 2016 Jun 10;95(23): e96d5. PMID: 25761173; PMCID: PMC4602475.

70. Shin WY, An MJ, Im NG, et al. Changes in Blood Glucose Level After Steroid Injection for Musculoskeletal Pain in Patients With Diabetes. Ann Rehabil Med 2020;44(2):117–24.

71. Ford LT, DeBender J. Tendon rupture after local steroid injection. South Med J 1979;72(7):827–30.

72. Fawi HMT, Hossain M, Matthews TJW. The incidence of flare reaction and short-term outcome following steroid injection in the shoulder. Shoulder Elbow 2017; 9(3):188–94.

73. Lubowitz JH, Brand JC, Rossi MJ. Preoperative Shoulder Corticosteroid Injection Is Associated With Revision After Primary Rotator Cuff Repair. Arthroscopy 2019;35(3):693–4.

74. Chevalier X. Acide hyaluronique dans la gonarthrose : mécanismes d'action. In: Chevalier X, editor. Injection d'acide hyaluronique et arthrose. Paris: Masson; 2005. p. 9–39.

75. Vannabouathong C, Bhandari M, Bedi A, et al. Nonoperative Treatments for Knee Osteoarthritis: An Evaluation of Treatment Characteristics and the Intra-Articular Placebo Effect: A Systematic Review. JBJS Rev 2018;6(7):e5.

76. Penning LI, de Bie RA, Walenkamp GH. The effectiveness of injections of hyaluronic acid or corticosteroid in patients with subacromial impingement: a three-arm randomised controlled trial. J Bone Joint Surg Br 2012;94(9): 1246–52.

77. Hsieh LF, Lin YJ, Hsu WC, et al. Comparison of the corticosteroid injection and hyaluronate in the treatment of chronic subacromial bursitis: A randomized controlled trial. Clin Rehabil 2021;35(9):1305–16.

78. Shakeri H, Keshavarz R, Arab AM, et al. Clinical effectiveness of kinesiological taping on pain and pain-free shoulder range of motion in patients with shoulder impingement syndrome: a randomized, double blinded, placebo-controlled trial. Int J Sports Phys Ther 2013;8(6):800–10.

79. Gebremariam L, Hay EM, van der Sande R, et al. Subacromial impingement syndrome–effectiveness of physiotherapy and manual therapy. Br J Sports Med 2014;48(16):1202–8.

80. Ellman H. Arthroscopic subacromial decompression: analysis of one- to three-year results. Arthroscopy 1987;3:173–81.

81. Davis AD, Kakar S, Moros C, et al. Arthroscopic versus open acromioplasty: a meta-analysis. Am J Sports Med 2010;38(3):613–8.

82. Dorrestijn O, Stevens M, Winters JC, et al. Conservative or surgical treatment for subacromial impingement syndrome? A systematic review. J Shoulder Elbow Surg 2009;18:652–60.
83. Colman WW, Kelkar R, Flatow EL, et al. The Effect of Anterior Acromioplasty on Rotator Cuff Contact: An Experimental and Computer Simulation. JSES 1996;5(2):2.
84. Heyworth BE, Williams RJ 3rd. Internal impingement of the shoulder. Am J Sports Med 2009;37(5):1024–37.
85. Meister K, Buckley B, Batts J. The posterior impingement sign: diagnosis of rotator cuff and posterior labral tears secondary to internal impingement in overhand athletes. Am J Orthop (Belle Mead Nj) 2004;33(8):412–5.
86. Davidson PA, ElAttrache NS, Jobe CM, et al. Rotator cuff and posterior-superior glenoid labrum injury associated with increased glenohumeral motion: a new site of impingement. J Shoulder Elbow Surg 1995;4(5):384–90.
87. Edelson G, Teitz C. Internal impingement in the shoulder. J Shoulder Elbow Surg 2000;9(4):308–15.
88. Paley KJ, Jobe FW, Pink MM, et al. Arthroscopic findings in the overhand throwing athlete: evidence for posterior internal impingement of the rotator cuff. Arthroscopy 2000;16(1):35–40.
89. Bennett GE. Elbow and shoulder lesions of baseball players. Am J Surg 1959; 98:484–92.
90. Giaroli EL, Major NM, Higgins LD. MRI of internal impingement of the shoulder. AJR Am J roentgenology 2005;185(4):925–9.
91. Fessa CK, Peduto A, Linklater J, et al. Posterosuperior glenoid internal impingement of the shoulder in the overhead athlete: pathogenesis, clinical features and MR imaging findings. J Med Imaging Radiat Oncol 2015;59(2):182–7.
92. Walch G, Boileau P, Noel E, et al. Impingement of the deep surface of the supraspinatus tendon on the posterosuperior glenoid rim: An arthroscopic study. J Shoulder Elbow Surg 1992;1(5):238–45.
93. Andrews JR, Broussard TS, Carson WG. Arthroscopy of the shoulder in the management of partial tears of the rotator cuff: a preliminary report. Arthroscopy 1985;1(2):117–22.
94. Levitz CL, Dugas J, Andrews JR. The use of arthroscopic thermal capsulorrhaphy to treat internal impingement in baseball players. Arthroscopy 2001;17(6): 573–7.
95. Yoneda M, Nakagawa S, Hayashida K, et al. Arthroscopic removal of symptomatic Bennett lesions in the shoulders of baseball players: arthroscopic Bennettplasty. Am J Sports Med 2002;30(5):728–36.
96. Riand N, Levigne C, Renaud E, et al. Results of derotational humeral osteotomy in posterosuperior glenoid impingement. Am J Sports Med 1998;26(3):453–9.
97. Freehill MQ. Coracoid impingement: diagnosis and treatment. J Am Acad Orthop Surg 2011;19(4):191–7. PMID: 21464212.
98. Gerber C, Terrier F, Zehnder R, et al. The subcoracoid space. An anatomic study. Clin Orthop Relat Res 1987;215:132–8. PMID: 3802629.
99. Osti L, Soldati F, Del Buono A, et al. Subcoracoid impingement and subscapularis tendon: is there any truth? Muscles Ligaments Tendons J 2013;3(2):101–5.
100. Dines D.M., Warren R.F., Inglis A.E., et al., The coracoid impingement syndrome, J Bone Joint Surg, 72 (2), 1990, 314–316.
101. Friedman RJ, Bonutti PM, Genez B. Cine magnetic resonance imaging of the subcoracoid region. Orthopedics 1998;21(5):545–8.

102. Giaroli EL, Major NM, Lemley DE, et al. Coracohumeral interval imaging in sub-coracoid impingement syndrome on MRI. AJR Am J Roentgenol 2006;186(1): 242–6.
103. Kleist KD, Freehill MQ, Hamilton L, et al. Computed tomography analysis of the coracoid process and anatomic structures of the shoulder after arthroscopic coracoid decompression: a cadaveric study. J Shoulder Elbow Surg 2007; 16(2):245–50.
104. Neer CS 2nd, Welsh RP. The shoulder in sports. Orthop Clin North Am 1977; 8(3):583–91.
105. Tibone JE, Jobe FW, Kerlan RK, et al. Shoulder impingement syndrome in ath-letes treated by an anterior acromioplasty. Clin Orthop Relat Res 1985;198: 134–40.

Nonoperative Treatment of Rotator Cuff Tears

Rebecca N. Dickinson, PT, DPT, OCS*, John E. Kuhn, MS, MD

KEYWORDS

- Rotator cuff tear • Conservative management • Nonoperative treatment
- Rehabilitation • Physical therapy

KEY POINTS

- Rotator cuff tears are very common, and prevalence increases with age.
- Best clinical examination includes a cluster of tests to determine rotator cuff involvement including lag signs.
- Rehabilitation or physical therapy has been shown to be an effective conservative treatment of rotator cuff tears with best outcomes seen in partial thickness tears, degenerative nontraumatic full-thickness tears, and massive irreparable tears.
- Tear progression happens in approximately 50% of full-thickness tears, but it is unclear in what circumstances the progression of tear correlates with the progression of pain and dysfunction.

INTRODUCTION/BACKGROUND/PREVALENCE

Rotator cuff tears can be described by the mechanism of injury as acute (or a traumatic—the result of an event with enough energy to cause immediate failure of an intact rotator cuff), acute on chronic (a preexisting rotator cuff tear enlarges after a traumatic event) or chronic (where no history of injury is present, and the tear is likely degenerative in nature). Rotator cuff tears can further be classified by anatomic severity as partial thickness or full-thickness tears. Full-thickness tears are further defined as small (<1 cm), medium (1 to 3 cm) large (3 to 5 cm), and massive (>5 cm). Prevalence of rotator cuff tears increases with age in both symptomatic and asymptomatic populations, and it has been estimated that approximately 10% of people aged 20 years or less have tears, increasing to 62% in those 80 years or older.[1] This information suggests that for many, rotator cuff degeneration is a natural aging process and that rotator cuff tears are quite often asymptomatic.[1,2]

[a] Vanderbilt Orthopedics Nashville, 1215 21 Street Avenue South, Suite 3200, Medical Center East, South Tower, Nashville, TN 37232, USA
* Corresponding author.
E-mail address: Rebecca.Dickinson@vumc.org
Twitter: @rndickinson (R.N.D.)

Phys Med Rehabil Clin N Am 34 (2023) 335–355
https://doi.org/10.1016/j.pmr.2022.12.002
1047-9651/23/© 2022 Elsevier Inc. All rights reserved.

These data suggest that rotator cuff tears frequently do not cause pain and disability. As such "It is important to be sure that operative interventions for the rotator cuff are a wise investment of hope, an effective use of resources, and worth the small but real risk of iatrogenic harm, the risk of medicalizing common symptoms, and the risk of interfering with the development of effective coping strategies."[1] Nonoperative treatment should be considered as an initial treatment in partial thickness tears, some full-thickness tears (especially smaller and atraumatic tears), chronic tears in older ages, and irreparable tears with muscle changes that are irreversible.[3] Acute tears and tears with substantial functional loss and weakness may be better treated with surgery.[4,5]

The objectives of this article were to (1) review appropriate examination techniques to determine rotator cuff tear diagnoses, (2) review and understand the evidence behind nonoperative treatment of rotator cuff tears as compared with surgery, (3) review current concepts and interventions, both pharmacological and nonpharmacological, in nonoperative treatment of rotator cuff tears, and (4) discuss outcomes and complications of nonoperative treatment.

PATIENT EVALUATION OVERVIEW
Clinical Assessment: History

There are many known risk factors associated with rotator cuff tears and a thorough history is essential. Risk factors associated with rotator cuff tears include the history of trauma, hand dominance, age over 65 years, diabetes, smoking, cervical spine pathology, long-term alcohol consumption, hypertension, family history/genetics, hypercholesterolemia, weakness with external rotation or elevation, and night pain.[3,6–11] If the following three factors: (1) age 65 years or older, (2) night pain, and (3) weakness with external rotation are present, there is a high suspicion of a rotator cuff tear (positive predictive value of 93.1% and +LR of 9.8).[6]

Clinical Assessment: Physical Examination

There are several physical examination tests that have been used to try to identify rotator cuff tears (**Table 1**)[12–14] (**Figs. 1–4**). Evidence for clinical special tests to detect rotator cuff tears is difficult to analyze, as many studies bring significant bias, decreased quality, and a range of severity in rotator cuff tear anatomy and symptoms. Clinical tests cannot differentiate a partial thickness or small full-thickness tear from subacromial pain syndrome without tear.[15,16] Lag signs (see **Figs. 2** and **4**) are helpful to identify larger full-thickness tears of the rotator cuff and are helpful when present, but because the negative likelihood ratio is not great, the absence of a lag sign cannot rule out a rotator cuff tear. In fact, it is difficult for any specific physical examination test to rule in or rule out rotator cuff tear.[17] A better choice is a cluster of physical examination tests that have shown higher odds or likelihood ratios, sensitivity, specificity, and/or positive predictive values. The combination of a positive painful arc, drop-arm sign (see **Fig. 1**), and weakness with infraspinatus muscle testing (aka resisted external rotation test) has been shown to have a 91% posttest probability for full-thickness tears.[15] The combination of the resisted external rotation test and the Patte sign (see **Fig. 3**) has been shown to have the highest correlation with intraoperative findings of infraspinatus tears.[16]

It is important to look for physical examination findings that can be addressed with nonoperative treatment that have been associated with symptomatic rotator cuff tears. Scapular dyskinesis, degrees of active abduction range of motion, strength of flexion and abduction, increased activity of the trapezius, and decreased activity of the deltoid have all been associated with symptomatic atraumatic full-thickness rotator cuff tears.[18,19]

Table 1
Special physical examination tests to identify larger full-thickness rotator cuff tears[15-17]

Test	Drop Arm Test (see Fig. 1)	External Rotation Lag Sign (see Fig. 2)	Hornblower's Sign (see Fig. 3)	Internal Rotation Lag Sign (see Fig. 4)
Performance description	The patient's arm is passively elevated to 90° in full external rotation, the patient is asked to slowly lower arm when support is removed, positive test is a sudden drop of the arm uncontrolled by the patient	The patient's elbow is passively flexed to 90° with the shoulder elevated to 20° in the scapular plane and near full external rotation, patient is asked to hold this position, a positive test is the sudden drop or inability to maintain this position, amount of lag can be measured by supporting the elbow and asking patient to hold external rotation and measuring the amount of drop	The patient's arm is elevated to 90° in the scapular plane with elbow flexed to 90, the patient is asked to create force into external rotation against manual resistance, the test is positive if the patient is unable to generate force	The patient's arm is placed in maximal internal rotation with the dorsum of the hand on the lumbar region of the spine, the examiner holds the wrist and elbow and extension the shoulder about 20°, the patient is asked to hold this position as the examiner releases the wrist but holds the elbow, positive test is the inability to hold the wrist away from the back
Tendon, specificity (SP), and sensitivity (SN)	Supraspinatus and infraspinatus SN 44, SP 98	Infraspinatus SN 69–98, SP 98	Infraspinatus SN 21, SP 92 Teres Minor SN 95, SN 92	Subscapularis SN 97, SP 96

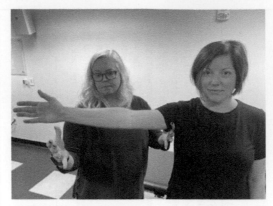

Fig. 1. Drop arm test (see **Table 1** for description of technique).

Clinical Assessment: Radiology

Imaging represents the most accurate way to identify rotator cuff tears. Plain radiographs may be helpful in large tears, as the humeral head may migrate superiorly. The acromiohumeral interval should be filled with supraspinatus tendon and an interval <6 mm is suggestive of a rotator cuff tear.[20,21] In addition, on a true AP of the glenohumeral joint (Grashey view) an arch exists spanning the medial humerus to the axillary border of the scapula (aka Shenton's line of the Shoulder or Moloney's Line). If this arch is disrupted by a superiorly migrated humeral head, this suggests a large rotator cuff tear is present.

MRI, MRI arthrography, and Ultrasound represent the most used imaging technique to identify rotator cuff tears. All of these techniques are very sensitive (.90, .90, .91 respectively), specific (.93, .95, .93), with very high + Likelihood Ratios (12.9, 18.0, 13.0) and very low -Likelihood Ratios (0.1, 0.1, 0.1).[22] Of the three tests, MRI is used more commonly, whereas ultrasound is more cost-effective but may require extensive training to reach optimal accuracy.[23]

PHARMACOLOGIC OR MEDICAL TREATMENT OPTIONS

Medications may be helpful to treat patients with symptomatic rotator cuff tears. Nonsteroidal Anti-Inflammatory Drugs are often prescribed for shoulder pain. Meta-analyses show these medications are effective in treating pain in the short term, but

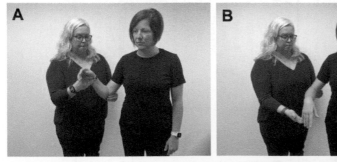

Fig. 2. (A) External rotation lag sign position (see **Table 1** for description of technique). (B) Positive ER lag sign.

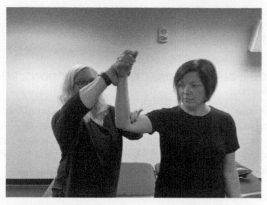

Fig. 3. Horn blower's sign (Patte test) (see **Table 1** for description of technique).

do not seem to improve function.[24] The use of opioids for chronic pain is not recommended; however, the use of opioids for treating rotator cuff symptoms seems higher than expected with up to 20.6% of patients with rotator cuff diagnoses receiving at least one opioid or benzodiazepine prescription at a large heath care center, and, of these, 21% had at least one risk factor for prescription misuse.[25]

Injectable corticosteroids are also commonly used to treat shoulder pain and rotator cuff disease. Most studies show these medications may provide short-term reduction in pain and improvement in function (3 to 6 weeks), but not long-term benefit compared with placebo (>24 weeks).[26–28] When compared with oral nonsteroidal anti-inflammatory drug (NSAIDs), injections of corticosteroids showed no significant advantage.[27]

Care must be taken as preoperative corticosteroid injections are correlated with an increased risk of revision rotator cuff surgery in a temporal and dose-dependent manner. If one is considering surgery, injections should be avoided and if an injection is given, surgery should be delayed at least six weeks to mitigate this risk.[29]

Platelet-rich plasma (PRP) has been studied as an injectable nonoperative treatment of rotator cuff disease. Systematic reviews suggest these can be effective in treating pain related to rotator cuff tendinosis and partial rotator cuff tears.[30] The effect

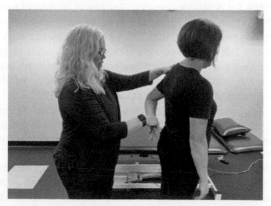

Fig. 4. Internal rotation lag sign (see **Table 1** for description of technique).

may last substantially longer than injectable corticosteroids.[26] As there are many variations in PRP preparation, there is substantial heterogeneity in the systematic reviews and the optimal PRP preparation is yet unknown.

NONPHARMACOLOGIC INTERVENTIONAL TREATMENT OPTIONS: REHABILITATION
Partial Thickness Tears

As mentioned previously, it is difficult to discern between partial thickness rotator cuff tears and subacromial pain syndrome/subacromial impingement. Nonsurgical treatment including physical therapy is suggested for partial thickness tears due to low evidence of progression of tear severity.[31] Treatment of partial thickness tears should follow guidelines for subacromial pain as described previously.

Full-thickness Tears

There is significant evidence supporting the first-line use of conservative treatment (including physical therapy and exercises) for managing atraumatic or degenerative full-thickness rotator cuff tears. To date, there are three randomized controlled trials comparing surgical versus nonoperative treatment of rotator cuff tears[32–34] (**Table 2**). There are also several large prospective cohort studies demonstrating successful treatment of rotator cuff tears nonoperatively[35–37] (**Table 3**). It is generally estimated that conservative treatment is effective in approximately 70% to 75% of patients as measured by avoiding surgical intervention. Interestingly, the MOON Shoulder Group identified low patient expectations regarding physical therapy as the most important variable to predict the need for surgery, whereas symptom severity or anatomic severity had little effect on the need for surgery.[38] Another group reported that patients who had higher pain or functional disturbances more than 10 years after nonoperative treatment were significantly younger than the rest of the cohort (54 years of age vs 64).[37] Although two of the randomized controlled trials report better pain and functional outcomes in the surgical group,[32,33] it is unclear how to determine which or how many patients would find this difference worth the risk, time lost from work and activities, and cost of surgical intervention given that up to 75% of patients treated conservatively are satisfied enough to not require surgery.[35–37]

It is also important to consider that studies have shown anywhere from a 20% to 94% rate of recurrent defects after surgical repair of a torn rotator cuff.[39–43] For open repairs, Harryman and colleagues[39] reported recurrent defects were seen in 20% of patients with only supraspinatus repairs, 43% for supraspinatus plus infraspinatus tears, and 68% for 3 tendon repairs. Boileau et al. found recurrent defects in 29% of patients after arthroscopic repair of full-thickness supraspinatus tears.[43] Interestingly several studies have shown that patient-reported outcomes are the same for patients whose repairs failed when compared with those whose repairs healed. But it is notable that in patients whose repairs healed, better strength was observed.[44,45] These data make it difficult to determine what is responsible for the improvements in pain and function seen after surgical rotator cuff repair.

In the literature, a wide variety of exercise interventions are used in nonoperative management of rotator cuff repairs. Another common parameter to consider is the duration and frequency of formal physical therapy and when a home exercise program will be sufficient treatment.

The studies included in **Tables 2** and **3** provide limited information regarding the specific exercise guidelines used. Kukkonen and colleagues[34] report their patients were educated in a home exercise program by a physical therapist in one visit. The first 6 weeks focused on glenohumeral range of motion and active scapular retraction,

Table 2
Randomized controlled trials comparing surgical and conservative treatment

	Moosmayer et al,[32] 2019	Kukkonen et al,[34] 2021	Lambers Heerspink et al,[33] 2015
N = (number of patients)	103	180	56
Follow-up years (% follow-up)	10 (88%)	5 (83%)	1 (80%)
Tear size included	Full-thickness not exceeding 3 cm	Atraumatic, symptomatic, isolated full-thickness supraspinatus tears in patients over 55	Degenerative full-thickness
Outcomes measures	Constant score; the self-report section of the American Shoulder and Elbow Surgeons Score; Short Form 36 Health Survey; measurement of pain, strength, and pain-free mobility of the shoulder	Constant score; visual analog score for pain; patient satisfaction	Constant score; visual analog scale for pain; visual analog scale for disability
Conclusion	At 10 years, the differences in outcomes between primary tendon repair and physiotherapy had increased, with better results for primary tendon repair	Operative treatment is no better than conservative treatment in small, nontraumatic, single-tendon supraspinatus tears in patients older than 55. Operative treatment does not protect against degeneration of the glenohumeral joint or cuff arthropathy. Conservative treatment is reasonable for initial treatment of these tears.	No differences in functional outcomes in Constant scores at 1 year. Significant differences in pain and disabilities were observed in favor of surgical treatment.

Table 3
Prospective cohort studies of conservative treatment of atraumatic rotator cuff tears

	Kijima et al,[37] 2012	Boorman et al,[36] 2018	Kuhn (MOON) et al,[35] 2013
N = (number of patients)	103 shoulders	104	452
Follow-up years (% follow-up)	13 (63%)	5 (84%)	2 (84%)
Tear size included	Rotator cuff tears by MRI (did not report size or traumatic vs atraumatic)	Chronic, full-thickness tears of supraspinatus or infraspinatus	Atraumatic, full-thickness tears
Outcomes measures	Japanese Orthopedic Association shoulder scoring system	Successful defined as no surgery needed vs failed as needing surgery, rotator cuff quality of life index	SF-12, ASES score, WORC index, SANE, Shoulder Activity Scale, cross-over to surgery
Conclusion	90% of patients had no or slight shoulder pain, 70% had no disturbance in activities of daily life, younger patient had more pain or disorder in daily life	75% were successfully treated with nonoperative management at 5 years, between 2 and 5 years, only 3 crossed over to surgery indicating most that were successful at 2 years remain so at 5 years	Nonoperative treatment affective in 75% of patient and most who crossed over to surgery did so between 6 and 12 weeks, few had surgery between 3 and 24 months

followed by a second 6 weeks of static and dynamic exercises for scapular and glenohumeral muscle function.[34] After 12 weeks, the patients increased resistance and strength for up to 6 months.[34] Moosemayer and colleagues[46] included in-person treatment sessions for 40 minutes each averaging twice a week for 12 weeks, with the possibility of lesser frequency visits throughout the following 6 to 12 weeks. This protocol was described as focusing on upper quarter posture and restoring scapulothoracic and glenohumeral muscular control and stability.[46] The cohorts by Kijima and colleagues[37] and Boorman and colleagues[36] both report including stretching and strengthening exercises but do not include specific on exercises are frequency and duration. Kuhn and colleagues[35] published their MOON Shoulder physical therapy protocol in detail and can be found at the following link: https://www.ncbi.nlm.nih.gov/pmc/articles/PMC3748251/

The MOON protocol includes flexibility and range of motion exercises that are performed daily and strengthening exercises that are performed three to four times a week with resistance that causes only minimal discomfort.[35] Rehabilitation after rotator cuff tear is obviously not focused on treating pathology, but more so on modifiable impairments including strength, range of motion, and motor control that are considered to affect pain and function.[47] In a clinical review, Edwards and colleagues[47] describe key evidence-based concepts; and in **Table 4** the authors suggested guidelines for an exercise-based protocol for conservative management of rotator cuff tears.

Glenohumeral range of motion is needed for best motor planning.[47] Therefore, exercises should be given to restore any range of motion deficits. **Figs. 5** and **6** show some common range of motion exercises.

Scapular movement has been shown to be affected by soft tissue tightness along with pain, altered motor control, strength imbalances and posture,[47,48] and specifically pectoralis minor and posterior glenohumeral capsular tightness have been associated with scapular dyskinesis.[49] Mobility of these two structures should be assessed and proper mobility exercises (**Figs. 7–9**) should be given for any deficits.

Suboptimal scapular movement control, or scapulohumeral rhythm, can have effects on rotator cuff strength and loading. In patients with rotator cuff-related pain, the serratus anterior and upper, middle, and lower trapezius are often seen to have changes in activation patterns and strength, specifically decreased or late activation of the serratus anterior and lower and middle trapezius and possibly hyperactivation of the upper trapezius.[47,49] **Figs. 10–12** are examples of common exercises given more strength and movement coordination patterns in these muscles suggested in the literature.[50,51]

The rotator cuff muscles are important to maintain the centering of the humeral head in the glenoid and a disruption of these muscles could cause elevation of the humeral head into the coracoacromial arch. But there is some evidence that there is some redundancy in the mechanism.[52] Hawkes and colleagues[52] showed increased activity of the scapular stabilizers, elbow flexors, latissimus dorsi and teres major in shoulders with rotator cuff tears to help balance the pull of the deltoid on the glenohumeral joint. Therefore, it is important to strengthen any remaining intact portions of the rotator cuff, but also consider mechanisms that can compensate for the deficient portions when developing a rehabilitation program.[47]

Massive, Irreparable Tears

In the literature, there have been several identified ways to classify rotator cuff tears. Goutallier and colleagues[53] introduced a system based on the amount of fatty infiltration in the torn cuff muscles and Patte and colleagues[54] described a classification

Table 4
Evidence-based exercise protocol for the conservative management of rotator cuff tears

Phase	Goals	Exercises	Dose	Progression

Range of motion (ROM)	1. Improve glenohumeral motions (forward flexion, abduction and external rotation)
	2. Improve shoulder and thoracic posture
		• Passive ROM (PROM)
		  ○ Forward flexion, internal/external rotation
		  ○ Pendulum (see **Fig. 2**)
		• Posture
		  ○ Postural education
		  ○ Scapula setting exercises
		• Active-assisted ROM (AAROM
		  ○ Wand exercises: elevation, abduction, adduction, internal/external rotation (see **Fig. 3**)
		  ○ Pulley-assisted elevation
		• Active ROM (AROM)
		  ○ Wall slides
			3 × 15 reps, daily	• ROM should begin with PROM and pendulum exercises progressing to AAROM and AROM as comfort dictates

Flexibility	1. Improve flexibility and reduce tightness of anterior and posterior capsule	• Anterior capsule (pectoralis minor) stretch
		  ○ Supine bear hugs
		  ○ Door frame stretch (see **Fig. 6**)
		• Posterior capsule stretch
		  ○ Cross-body stretch (see **Fig. 5**)
		  ○ Towel stretch
		• Upper trapezius stretch
			5 × 30 s stretches, daily	N/A

| Strengthening | 1. Improve strength of the scapular stabilizing muscles and dynamic scapular control
2. Improve strength of the anterior deltoid for shoulder elevation
3. Improve active external rotation strength | • Isometric low rows (see **Fig. 7**)
• Scapula retraction/rows
  ○ Prone scapula retractions (squeezes), prone shoulder extension (see **Fig. 9**)
  ○ Bent over rows, seated/standing (elastic resistance)
• Scapula protractions/presses
  ○ Supine scapula protraction
  ○ Upright wall scapula protractions/retractions, wall push-ups
  ○ Quadruped scapula protractions
  ○ Standing scapula presses with elastic resistance
• Anterior deltoid strengthening
  ○ Isometric deltoid contractions
  ○ Should flexion; supine (see **Fig. 10**), inverted (see **Fig. 11**) and standing (see **Fig. 12**)
• External Rotation
  ○ Standing 0° abduction with elastic resistance | 3 × 15 reps per exercise, 3 to 4 times per week | • Strengthening is undertaken within limits of pain
• Increase volume and load, as comfort, strength and tolerance dictate
• Patients exceeding appropriate discomfort level should reduce the level of resistance |

(continued on next page)

Table 4
(continued)

Phase	Goals	Exercises	Dose	Progression
		○ Side lying with dumbbell (see **Fig. 8**) • Internal Rotation ○ Standing 0° abduction with elastic resistance ○ Side lying with dumbbell		
Strengthening/proprioception (advanced)	1. Advance strengthening of the scapular stabilizers 2. Advance strengthening of the rotator cuff 3. Introduce work/sport-specific exercises	• Scapula protractions/presses ○ Upright Fitball push-ups, push-ups on ground ○ Standing cable press ○ Dynamic bug exercise • External rotation ○ Seated and standing 90° abduction (dumbbell and elastic resistance) ○ External rotation 90° prone horizontal abduction • Internal rotation ○ Standing 90° abduction (elastic resistance)	3 × 15 reps per exercise, 3 to 4 times per week	• Strengthening is undertaken within limits of pain • Increase volume and load, as comfort, strength and tolerance dictate • Patients exceeding appropriate discomfort level should reduce the level of resistance

(Copyright © 2016 Int J Sports Phys Ther. Apr 2016;11(2):279-301. Exercise Rehabilitation In The Non-operative Management Of Rotator Cuff Tears: A Review Of The Literature. Authors: Edwards P, Ebert J, Joss B, Bhabra G, Ackland T, Wang A.)

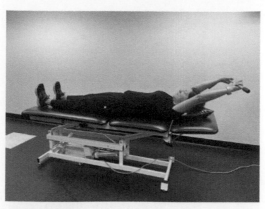

Fig. 5. Supine active assisted flexion.

system to quantify the amount of retraction from the greater tuberosity in the torn tendons. It has been shown that chronic rotator cuff tears involving 2 or more tendons with significant retraction (Patte grade 3) and Goutallier grade 3 or 4 fatty infiltration are less likely to respond well to surgical repair.[43,53,55–57] For patients whose tears meet these criteria, nonoperative management including physical therapy, is often the first line of treatment.

In a systematic review in 2021, Shepet and colleagues[58] identified 10 level III and IV studies addressing clinical outcomes of nonoperative treatment of massive, irreparable rotator cuff tears; no level I or II studies were identified. The authors found that nonoperative treatment was reported as successful in a range from 32% to 100% of cases. In these studies, poor outcomes were associated with abduction and external rotation strength <3/5, muscular atrophy, superior migration of the humeral head, decreased glenohumeral passive range of motion, glenohumeral osteoarthritis, active forward flexion <50°, anterior cuff tears, subscapularis tears, and lack of teres minor hypertrophy.[59–62] The most included range of motion exercises were into forward flexion and external rotation.[58] Other commonly found interventions found in this systematic review included an anterior deltoid program that progresses from supine to upright, deltoid and teres minor strengthening, and supervised physical

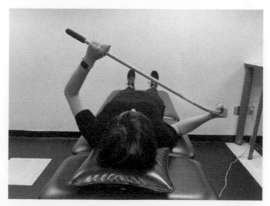

Fig. 6. Supine active assisted external rotation.

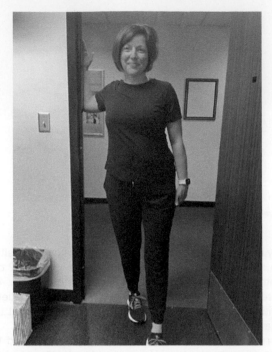

Fig. 7. Pectoralis minor door stretch.

therapy up to 8 to 12 weeks.[58] Shepet and colleagues[58] went on to publish a detailed synthesized protocol along with this systematic review and contains specifics of the suggested guidelines.

TREATMENT RESISTANCE/COMPLICATIONS

Tear progression could be considered a possible complication of nonoperative treatment of cuff tears. It is reasonable to consider the possibility that a repairable rotator cuff tear could progress to a massive irreparable tear and that the long-term outcomes

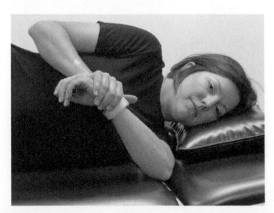

Fig. 8. Sleeper stretch.

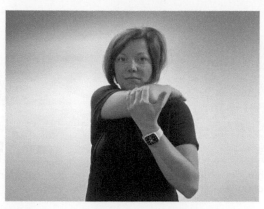

Fig. 9. Cross-body stretch.

may be better in someone who decided on earlier surgical intervention. Unfortunately, the evidence is unclear on which patients will have a progression of tear size and in which patients this progression may or may not cause a progression or new onset of symptoms.

A significant number of partial and full-thickness rotator cuff tears will progress in size over time. Keener and colleagues[63] looked at patients with asymptomatic rotator cuff tears in patients with pain and rotator cuff disease in the contralateral shoulder. One hundred and eighteen subjects with full-thickness tears, 56 with partial thickness tears, and 50 controls were followed for a median of 5.1 years. Tears enlarged greater than 5 millimeters (mm) in 49% of shoulders (61% of full-thickness tears, 44% of partial thickness tears, and 14% of controls) and median time to enlargement was 2.8 years, with tear enlargement being associated with new onset of pain.[63] Moosmayer and colleagues[64] followed 49 patients over 8.8 years with symptomatic small to medium full-thickness primarily treated with physical therapy, with 37 being re-evaluated by MRI. Mean tear size increased 8.3 mm and 4.5 mm in the anterior/posterior and medial/lateral planes respectively.[64] Jung and colleagues[65] looked at MRI's in 48 patients following conservative treatment with mean follow-up of 22 months. Anterior posterior tear progression was seen in 54% of patients and medial lateral

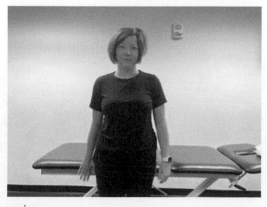

Fig. 10. Low row exercise.

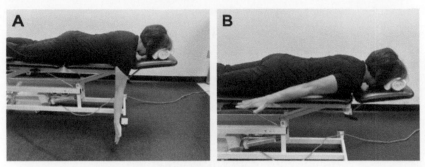

Fig. 11. (*A*) Prone shoulder extension exercise starting position. (*B*) Prone shoulder extension exercise finish position.

progression in 41%, with increase being defined as greater than 5 mm, with severe infraspinatus atrophy as the independent risk factor for tear enlargement.[65] Although Keener and colleagues[63] found an association between tear enlargement and an onset of symptoms, the MOON (Multi-Center Orthopedic Outcomes Network) shoulder group found that duration of symptoms did not correlate with severity of rotator cuff disease or tear size[66] and patients who cross over to surgery from conservative care are more influenced by low expectations regarding physical therapy than anatomic features of the rotator cuff tear.[38] More studies are needed to determine if tear progression, which happens in at least half of full-thickness tears in the above studies, correlates to increased symptoms, and what characteristics are risk factors for the onset or increase in symptoms.

Other possible barriers to positive outcomes are psychosocial factors. In a systematic review looking at psychosocial factors associated with outcomes in patients with rotator cuff tears by Coronado and colleagues,[67] the authors found weak to moderate associations for emotional or mental health with function and disability and pain. Lower emotional or mental health was associated with lower physical function and higher pain and disability at initial evaluation for rotator cuff tear and patient expectations were associated with patient reported outcomes after treatment.[67] It is currently unclear how clinicians can affect these factors, when referral should be made to other specialties in this area of expertise, and what effects intervention would have on outcomes.

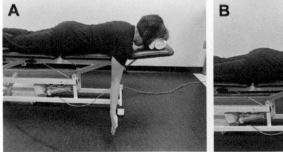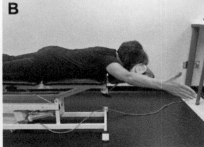

Fig. 12. (*A*) Prone scaption exercise starting position. (*B*) Prone scaption exercise finish position.

SUMMARY/DISCUSSION/FUTURE DIRECTIONS

Conservative treatment has been shown to be effective in many patients with rotator cuff tears. Nonsurgical care is often the first line of treatment of partial thickness tears, degenerative nontraumatic full-thickness tears, and massive irreparable tears.

Suggested future directions could include continuing to determine specific predictors for failure of nonoperative treatment of rotator cuff tears and better exploration of physical therapy parameters needed for success including supervision, frequency and duration, specific exercises and interventions along with dosing. Further information is also needed in what psychosocial factors affect outcomes in this population and how we can intervene to improve the factors that do affect positive outcomes in this patient population.

CLINICS CARE POINTS

- Prevalence of rotator cuff tears increases with age in both symptomatic and asymptomatic populations
- Approximately 10% of people aged 20 years or less have tears, increasing to 62% in those 80 years or older
- If all three factors of age 65 years or older, night pain, and weakness with external rotation are present, there is a high suspicion of a rotator cuff tear (positive predictive value of 93.1% and +LR of 9.8)
- Rehabilitation or physical therapy has been shown to be an effective conservative treatment of rotator cuff tears with best outcomes seen in partial thickness tears, degenerative nontraumatic full-thickness tears, and massive irreparable tears
- Physical therapy should include restoring range of motion, addressing any pectoralis minor or posterior capsule stiffness, and restoring motor control/strength to the scapula and rotator cuff

DISCLOSURE

R.N. Dickinson has no disclosures. J.E. Kuhn has no disclosures.

REFERENCES

1. Teunis T, Lubberts B, Reilly BT, et al. A systematic review and pooled analysis of the prevalence of rotator cuff disease with increasing age. J Shoulder Elbow Surg 2014;23(12):1913–21.
2. Reilly P, Macleod I, Macfarlane R, et al. Dead men and radiologists don't lie: a review of cadaveric and radiological studies of rotator cuff tear prevalence. Ann R Coll Surg Engl 2006;88(2):116–21.
3. Tashjian RZ. Epidemiology, natural history, and indications for treatment of rotator cuff tears. Clin Sports Med 2012;31(4):589–604.
4. Marx RG, Koulouvaris P, Chu SK, et al. Indications for surgery in clinical outcome studies of rotator cuff repair. Clin Orthop Relat Res 2009;467(2):450–6.
5. Oh LS, Wolf BR, Hall MP, et al. Indications for rotator cuff repair: a systematic review. Clin Orthop Relat Res 2007;455:52–63.
6. Litaker D, Pioro M, El Bilbeisi H, et al. Returning to the bedside: using the history and physical examination to identify rotator cuff tears. J Am Geriatr Soc 2000; 48(12):1633–7.

7. Yamamoto A, Takagishi K, Osawa T, et al. Prevalence and risk factors of a rotator cuff tear in the general population. J Shoulder Elbow Surg 2010;19(1):116–20.
8. Jeong J, Shin DC, Kim TH, et al. Prevalence of asymptomatic rotator cuff tear and their related factors in the Korean population. J Shoulder Elbow Surg 2017; 26(1):30–5.
9. Wang JY, Lin YR, Liaw CK, et al. Cervical spine pathology increases the risk of rotator cuff tear: a population-based cohort study. Orthop J Sports Med 2021; 9(12). 23259671211058726.
10. Passaretti D, Candela V, Venditto T, et al. Association between alcohol consumption and rotator cuff tear. Acta Orthop 2016;87(2):165–8.
11. Zhao J, Pan J, Zeng LF, et al. Risk factors for full-thickness rotator cuff tears: a systematic review and meta-analysis. EFORT Open Rev 2021;6(11):1087–96.
12. Hertel R, Ballmer FT, Lombert SM, et al. Lag signs in the diagnosis of rotator cuff rupture. J Shoulder Elbow Surg 1996;5(4):307–13.
13. Walch G, Boulahia A, Calderone S, et al. The 'dropping' and 'hornblower's' signs in evaluation of rotator-cuff tears. J Bone Joint Surg Br 1998;80(4):624–8.
14. Barth JR, Burkhart SS, De Beer JF. The bear-hug test: a new and sensitive test for diagnosing a subscapularis tear. Arthroscopy 2006;22(10):1076–84.
15. Park HB, Yokota A, Gill HS, et al. Diagnostic accuracy of clinical tests for the different degrees of subacromial impingement syndrome. J Bone Joint Surg Am 2005;87(7):1446–55.
16. Sgroi M, Loitsch T, Reichel H, et al. Diagnostic Value of Clinical Tests for Infraspinatus Tendon Tears. Arthroscopy 2019;35(5):1339–47.
17. Gismervik S, Drogset JO, Granviken F, et al. Physical examination tests of the shoulder: a systematic review and meta-analysis of diagnostic test performance. BMC Musculoskelet Disord 2017;18(1):41.
18. Harris JD, Pedroza A, Jones GL, Group MMOONS. Predictors of pain and function in patients with symptomatic, atraumatic full-thickness rotator cuff tears: a time-zero analysis of a prospective patient cohort enrolled in a structured physical therapy program. Am J Sports Med 2012;40(2):359–66.
19. Shinozaki N, Sano H, Omi R, et al. Differences in muscle activities during shoulder elevation in patients with symptomatic and asymptomatic rotator cuff tears: analysis by positron emission tomography. J Shoulder Elbow Surg 2014;23(3): e61–7.
20. Golding FC. The shoulder–the forgotten joint. Br J Radiol 1962;35:149–58.
21. Goutallier D, Le Guilloux P, Postel JM, et al. Acromio humeral distance less than six millimeter: its meaning in full-thickness rotator cuff tear. Orthop Traumatol Surg Res 2011;97(3):246–51.
22. Roy JS, Braën C, Leblond J, et al. Diagnostic accuracy of ultrasonography, MRI and MR arthrography in the characterisation of rotator cuff disorders: a systematic review and meta-analysis. Br J Sports Med 2015;49(20):1316–28.
23. Day M, Phil M, McCormack RA, et al. Physician training ultrasound and accuracy of diagnosis in rotator cuff tears. Bull Hosp Jt Dis 2013;74(3):207–11, 2016.
24. Boudreault J, Desmeules F, Roy JS, et al. The efficacy of oral non-steroidal anti-inflammatory drugs for rotator cuff tendinopathy: a systematic review and meta-analysis. J Rehabil Med 2014;46(4):294–306.
25. Gorbaty J, Odum SM, Wally MK, et al. Prevalence of Prescription Opioids for Nonoperative Treatment of Rotator Cuff Disease Is High. Arthrosc Sports Med Rehabil 2021;3(2):e373–9.
26. Lin MT, Chiang CF, Wu CH, et al. Comparative Effectiveness of Injection Therapies in Rotator Cuff Tendinopathy: A Systematic Review, Pairwise and Network

Meta-analysis of Randomized Controlled Trials. Arch Phys Med Rehabil 2019; 100(2):336–49.e15.

27. Buchbinder R, Green S, Youd JM. Corticosteroid injections for shoulder pain. Cochrane Database Syst Rev 2003;1:CD004016.

28. Mohamadi A, Chan JJ, Claessen FM, et al. Corticosteroid Injections Give Small and Transient Pain Relief in Rotator Cuff Tendinosis: A Meta-analysis. Clin Orthop Relat Res 2017;475(1):232–43.

29. Puzzitiello RN, Patel BH, Lavoie-Gagne O, et al. Corticosteroid Injections After Rotator Cuff Repair Improve Function, Reduce Pain, and Are Safe: A Systematic Review. Arthrosc Sports Med Rehabil 2022;4(2):e763–74.

30. Xiang XN, Deng J, Liu Y, et al. Conservative treatment of partial-thickness rotator cuff tears and tendinopathy with platelet-rich plasma: a systematic review and meta-analysis. Clin Rehabil 2021;35(12):1661–73.

31. Plancher KD, Shanmugam J, Briggs K, et al. Diagnosis and management of partial thickness rotator cuff tears: a comprehensive review. J Am Acad Orthop Surg 2021;29(24):1031–43.

32. Moosmayer S, Lund G, Seljom US, et al. At a 10-year follow-up, tendon repair is superior to physiotherapy in the treatment of small and medium-sized rotator cuff tears. J Bone Joint Surg Am 2019;101(12):1050–60.

33. Lambers Heerspink FO, van Raay JJ, Koorevaar RC, et al. Comparing surgical repair with conservative treatment for degenerative rotator cuff tears: a randomized controlled trial. J Shoulder Elbow Surg 2015;24(8):1274–81.

34. Kukkonen J, Ryösä A, Joukainen A, et al. Operative versus conservative treatment of small, nontraumatic supraspinatus tears in patients older than 55 years: over 5-year follow-up of a randomized controlled trial. J Shoulder Elbow Surg 2021;30(11):2455–64.

35. Kuhn JE, Dunn WR, Sanders R, et al. Effectiveness of physical therapy in treating atraumatic full-thickness rotator cuff tears: a multicenter prospective cohort study. J Shoulder Elbow Surg 2013;22(10):1371–9.

36. Boorman RS, More KD, Hollinshead RM, et al. What happens to patients when we do not repair their cuff tears? Five-year rotator cuff quality-of-life index outcomes following nonoperative treatment of patients with full-thickness rotator cuff tears. J Shoulder Elbow Surg 2018;27(3):444–8.

37. Kijima H, Minagawa H, Nishi T, et al. Long-term follow-up of cases of rotator cuff tear treated conservatively. J Shoulder Elbow Surg 2012;21(4):491–4.

38. Dunn WR, Kuhn JE, Sanders R, et al. 2013 Neer Award: predictors of failure of nonoperative treatment of chronic, symptomatic, full-thickness rotator cuff tears. J Shoulder Elbow Surg 2016;25(8):1303–11.

39. Harryman DT, Mack LA, Wang KY, et al. Repairs of the rotator cuff. Correlation of functional results with integrity of the cuff. J Bone Joint Surg Am 1991;73(7): 982–9.

40. Nho SJ, Brown BS, Lyman S, et al. Prospective analysis of arthroscopic rotator cuff repair: prognostic factors affecting clinical and ultrasound outcome. J Shoulder Elbow Surg 2009;18(1):13–20.

41. Cho NS, Rhee YG. The factors affecting the clinical outcome and integrity of arthroscopically repaired rotator cuff tears of the shoulder. Clin Orthop Surg 2009; 1(2):96–104.

42. Gusmer PB, Potter HG, Donovan WD, et al. MR imaging of the shoulder after rotator cuff repair. AJR Am J Roentgenol 1997;168(2):559–63.

43. Boileau P, Brassart N, Watkinson DJ, et al. Arthroscopic repair of full-thickness tears of the supraspinatus: does the tendon really heal? J Bone Joint Surg Am 2005;87(6):1229–40.

44. Slabaugh MA, Nho SJ, Grumet RC, et al. Does the literature confirm superior clinical results in radiographically healed rotator cuffs after rotator cuff repair? Arthroscopy 2010;26(3):393–403.

45. Russell RD, Knight JR, Mulligan E, et al. Structural integrity after rotator cuff repair does not correlate with patient function and pain: a meta-analysis. J Bone Joint Surg Am 2014;96(4):265–71.

46. Moosmayer S, Lund G, Seljom U, et al. Comparison between surgery and physiotherapy in the treatment of small and medium-sized tears of the rotator cuff: A randomised controlled study of 103 patients with one-year follow-up. J Bone Joint Surg Br 2010;92(1):83–91.

47. Edwards P, Ebert J, Joss B, et al. Exercise rehabilitation in the nonoperative management of rotator cuff tears: a review of the literature. Int J Sports Phys Ther 2016;11(2):279–301.

48. Ludewig PM, Reynolds JF. The association of scapular kinematics and glenohumeral joint pathologies. J Orthop Sports Phys Ther 2009;39(2):90–104.

49. Cools AM, Struyf F, De Mey K, et al. Rehabilitation of scapular dyskinesis: from the office worker to the elite overhead athlete. Br J Sports Med 2014;48(8):692–7.

50. Cools AM, Dewitte V, Lanszweert F, et al. Rehabilitation of scapular muscle balance: which exercises to prescribe? Am J Sports Med 2007;35(10):1744–51.

51. Kibler WB, Sciascia AD, Uhl TL, et al. Electromyographic analysis of specific exercises for scapular control in early phases of shoulder rehabilitation. Am J Sports Med 2008;36(9):1789–98.

52. Hawkes DH, Alizadehkhaiyat O, Kemp GJ, et al. Shoulder muscle activation and coordination in patients with a massive rotator cuff tear: an electromyographic study. J Orthop Res 2012;30(7):1140–6.

53. Goutallier D, Postel JM, Bernageau J, et al. Fatty muscle degeneration in cuff ruptures. Pre- and postoperative evaluation by CT scan. Clin Orthop Relat Res 1994;(304):78–83.

54. Patte D. Classification of rotator cuff lesions. Clin Orthop Relat Res 1990;(254):81–6.

55. Barry JJ, Lansdown DA, Cheung S, et al. The relationship between tear severity, fatty infiltration, and muscle atrophy in the supraspinatus. J Shoulder Elbow Surg 2013;22(1):18–25.

56. Tashjian RZ, Hung M, Burks RT, et al. Influence of preoperative musculotendinous junction position on rotator cuff healing using single-row technique. Arthroscopy 2013;29(11):1748–54.

57. Thomazeau H, Boukobza E, Morcet N, et al. Prediction of rotator cuff repair results by magnetic resonance imaging. Clin Orthop Relat Res 1997;344:275–83.

58. Shepet KH, Liechti DJ, Kuhn JE. Nonoperative treatment of chronic, massive irreparable rotator cuff tears: a systematic review with synthesis of a standardized rehabilitation protocol. J Shoulder Elbow Surg 2021;30(6):1431–44.

59. Vad VB, Warren RF, Altchek DW, et al. Negative prognostic factors in managing massive rotator cuff tears. Clin J Sport Med 2002;12(3):151–7.

60. Yian EH, Sodl JF, Dionysian E, et al. Anterior deltoid reeducation for irreparable rotator cuff tears revisited. J Shoulder Elbow Surg 2017;26(9):1562–5.

61. Collin PG, Gain S, Nguyen Huu F, et al. Is rehabilitation effective in massive rotator cuff tears? Orthop Traumatol Surg Res 2015;101(4 Suppl):S203–5.

62. Yoon TH, Kim SJ, Choi CH, et al. An intact subscapularis tendon and compensatory teres minor hypertrophy yield lower failure rates for nonoperative treatment of irreparable, massive rotator cuff tears. Knee Surg Sports Traumatol Arthrosc 2019;27(10):3240–5.
63. Keener JD, Galatz LM, Teefey SA, et al. A prospective evaluation of survivorship of asymptomatic degenerative rotator cuff tears. J Bone Joint Surg Am 2015; 97(2):89–98.
64. Moosmayer S, Gärtner AV, Tariq R. The natural course of nonoperatively treated rotator cuff tears: an 8.8-year follow-up of tear anatomy and clinical outcome in 49 patients. J Shoulder Elbow Surg 2017;26(4):627–34.
65. Jung W, Lee S, Hoon Kim S. The natural course of and risk factors for tear progression in conservatively treated full-thickness rotator cuff tears. J Shoulder Elbow Surg 2020;29(6):1168–76.
66. Unruh KP, Kuhn JE, Sanders R, et al. The duration of symptoms does not correlate with rotator cuff tear severity or other patient-related features: a cross-sectional study of patients with atraumatic, full-thickness rotator cuff tears. J Shoulder Elbow Surg 2014;23(7):1052–8.
67. Coronado RA, Seitz AL, Pelote E, et al. Are psychosocial factors associated with patient-reported outcome measures in patients with rotator cuff tears? A systematic review. Clin Orthop Relat Res 2018;476(4):810–29.

Postoperative Rehabilitation Following Rotator Cuff Repair

Taylor Swansen, MD, Melissa A. Wright, MD,
Anand M. Murthi, MD*

KEYWORDS

- Rotator cuff • Postoperative • Rotator cuff repair • Rehabilitation • Physical therapy

KEY POINTS

- It is important to individualize therapy based on repair integrity, tissue quality, and patient/host factors such as revision status and smoking history.
- The first stage of therapy focuses on allowing for anatomic rotator cuff healing while maintaining a passive range of motion.
- The second stage aims to protect the repair while reestablishing dynamic shoulder stability and developing full active and passive range of motion.
- The third stage aims to maintain shoulder range of motion while progressing with shoulder stabilization exercises and adding functional shoulder exercises.
- The fourth stage aims to restore full function strength and implement sport-specific training if necessary.

INTRODUCTION

Rotator cuff pathologic condition is a common cause of shoulder pain and dysfunction in patients across varying age groups. Although some patients and tear types may be successfully managed nonoperatively, rotator cuff repair has been shown to improve patient function and decrease pain.[1] Surgical treatment also helps to counteract the risk of tear progression, muscle atrophy, and further degenerative change in the setting of rotator cuff pathologic condition.

Postoperative rehabilitation including some type of physical therapy program is an integral part of a successful clinical outcome following a rotator cuff repair. Many studies have shown that active and passive range of motion, as well as strengthening exercises, reduces shoulder stiffness, and improves function following repair.[2]

Department of Orthopaedics, MedStar Union Memorial Hospital, 3333 North Calvert Street, Suite 400, Baltimore, MD 21218, USA
* Corresponding author.
E-mail address: amurthi14@hotmail.com

Phys Med Rehabil Clin N Am 34 (2023) 357–364
https://doi.org/10.1016/j.pmr.2022.12.003
1047-9651/23/© 2022 Elsevier Inc. All rights reserved.

Stiffness is common following rotator cuff tear and is related to patient age at the time of the repair as well as the preoperative level of stiffness.[3] However, retear is one of the most common complications following a repair. Although this has not been proven to be attributed to aggressive rehabilitation, retear rates may be up to 94% in larger tears.[4] Due to the potential risk of injury to the repair in the postoperative period, surgeons vary in the timing and intensity of postoperative exercises and the utilization of formal outpatient physical therapy versus a home surgeon-directed rehabilitation program.[2] Although the speed of surgeon-directed rehabilitation may vary based on repair characteristics, slower rehabilitation postoperatively has been shown not to increase rates of stiffness at 1 year.[5] Continued research on rehabilitation following rotator cuff repair will help surgeons refine protocols to optimize results, particularly the balance of preventing both tendon retear and stiffness. In our practice, we delay mobilization with a larger tear, in the setting of revision surgery needing graft augmentation, or with poor tissue quality.

CLINICAL CONSIDERATIONS

Rotator cuff tendon healing progresses through several well-described phases: the inflammatory phase (days 1–7), proliferative phase (days 7–21), and finally the maturation/remodeling phase (12–26 weeks).[6] The goal of an ideal postoperative rehabilitation protocol is to balance anatomic healing of the repair with shoulder mobility and strength. The overall rehabilitation process typically takes around 6 months and can be divided into 4 phases, which we highlight in this article. Most patients should expect minimal to no pain before they progress to the second phase of therapy, usually at around 6 weeks.[7] They should expect to achieve full range of motion and return to functional exercises at around 3 months as they enter phase 3. Full strength and endurance will take several more months to achieve.[7]

Several factors influence the likelihood that a rotator cuff repair will heal successfully, which a surgeon should consider when tailoring a rehabilitation protocol to the individual patient. Tear-related factors that influence healing include the size of tear, muscular atrophy, and retraction.[8] The location of the tear and presence of preoperative stiffness have also been found to influence healing rates, with isolated supraspinatus tears and presence of preoperative stiffness showing higher healing rates.[9,10] Tendon tissue quality and delamination also affect healing. Patient factors that influence healing include higher patient age, history of smoking, presence of diabetes mellitus or hyperlipidemia, and high body mass index.[11]

Home-directed physical therapy may be as effective as formal outpatient physical therapy following rotator cuff repair in some circumstances. Studies have shown no difference in patient outcomes between home exercises compared with formal physical therapy.[12,13] Due to concerns about patient compliance and the complexity of the rehabilitation process, many surgeons use formal physical therapy to help optimize patient outcomes. The number and frequency of therapy visits will vary by the patient and their needs but on average, patients will visit physical therapy from 12 to 28 times during their rehabilitation process.[13]

When using formal outpatient physical therapy, it is important for a surgeon to have good communication with the physical therapist to enhance the patient's rehabilitation process. Frequent communication can prevent damage to healing repairs and stiffness, which can delay return to full function. Including the operative report with the therapy protocol can help to enhance therapist understanding of the details of the repair and tissue quality, especially for more complex cases or revision cases. There are 4 standard phases in the rotator cuff repair rehabilitation process (**Table 1**). These

Table 1
Phases of physical therapy after rotator cuff repair

	Goals	Limitations	Exercises
Phase 1[a] Week 1–6	• Protect surgical repair • Restore range of motion • Decrease pain and inflammation • Emphasize home exercise program	• Wear a sling unless performing exercises • Passive-assisted or active-assisted motion only • External rotation in the scapular plane should not exceed 45°	• Passive and active assisted flexion, scaption, internal, and external rotation • Active wrist and elbow range of motion • Hand grip with putty • Pendulums • Shoulder isometrics at 0° and 45° abduction
Phase 2 Week 6–12	• Restore range of motion • Initiate active muscle contractions with a focus on regaining proper scapula-humeral rhythm • Training in joint proprioception	• No restrictions in flexion, elevation, or internal and external rotation in the scapular plane	• Phase 1 exercises • Internal rotation and posterior capsule stretches • Active range of motion exercises, progressed from supine to partial sitting to standing • Scapular strengthening with rows/shrugs/punches • Two-handed plyometrics
Phase 3 Week 12–14	• Restore full active range of motion • Progress strengthening and scapular stabilization exercises • Initiate more functional drills into the rehabilitation program	• Therapeutic exercises with a 7-lb maximum	• Range of motion exercises to maintain full range • Phase 2 exercises, increase intensity/sets/repetitions • Push-up progression • Theraband external rotation in the 90/90 position • Prone therapeutic exercises
Phase 4 Week 14–24	• Build full functional strength • Implement functional or sport specific training • Establish a progressive gym program	• None	• Phase 3 exercises • One-handed plyometric exercises • Eccentric rotator cuff strengthening • Large muscle exercises

[a] When biceps tenodesis is performed, no active range of motion of the elbow should be allowed during the first 3 wk after surgery. For larger tears, patients may be immobilized for up to 6 wk before initiating phases of therapy. In that case, Phase 1 should progress over 2 wk then continue to phase 2.

phases should be adjusted based on the size of the rotator cuff tear and the individual patient's progress.

Phase 1

In the first phase of rehabilitation protocol, the goal is to protect the surgical repair and to initiate range of motion. Emphasis on range of motion will prevent adhesions and increase circulation. In this phase, the aim is also to decrease pain and inflammation and emphasize the importance of a home exercise program. This phase occurs during week 1 to week 6 of recovery.

Baseline patient precautions include wearing a sling for 6 weeks unless otherwise instructed. Patients may remove the sling to perform exercises at home or under the supervision of a physical therapist. A sling with abduction pillow can be useful because the rotator cuff has better blood supply when the arm is held slightly away from the body. Alternatively, the patient can be counselled to use a towel roll under the arm while in a resting position. Sling immobilization may not be necessary for small to medium tears. Studies have shown that without sling immobilization, patients have earlier return of range of motion, although early mobilization has not been shown to affect long-term outcomes.[14] Slings are useful to protect the repair but they may increase the risk of early stiffness or exacerbate muscular weakness.[15] The risks and benefits of sling wear vary based on the patient and tear and the decision to recommend sling wear and the duration of sling wear may be determined by the treating surgeon.

Range of motion for the first phase should be passive and active-assisted only. Flexion and scaption may progress as tolerated, although patients with larger repairs should be counselled to progress slowly. Internal rotation in the scapular plane may progress as tolerated, and internal rotation behind the back may be assisted with towel stretches to tolerance, with the goal of reaching the same level as the contralateral shoulder. Internal rotation is often neglected due to limitations with passive-assisted and active-assisted joint motion, leading to posterior capsule stiffness and overall decreased motion. External rotation in the scapular plane should not exceed 45°. Active wrist and elbow range of motion should be encouraged. However, if a biceps tenodesis has been performed, no active range of motion of the elbow should be done during the first 3 weeks from surgery to protect the tenodesis.

Exercises in the first phase should focus on range of motion and maintaining scapular mechanics. Passive range of motion with pendulum exercises should be initiated early. Active assisted flexion, either supine or with a cane, may progress as tolerated. Seated or supine horizontal adduction may be used to stretch the posterior rotator cuff. At 3 to 4 weeks postoperatively, active-assisted external rotation at 0° and 45° of abduction may be initiated for smaller tears. Rope and pulley exercises in flexion and scaption may also be initiated at that time. Therapist-guided grade I-II glenohumeral and scapular mobilization and manual stretching may also be used during this time.

During the first 3 weeks of this phase, the patient should not work on active shoulder flexion or abduction. They may begin pain-free shoulder isometrics at 0° of abduction starting at week 2 at the earliest. Hand gripping exercises using putty may be used.

Patients should be counselled to use heat before therapy sessions. They should use ice following therapy sessions and as needed during the first phase of rehabilitation.

The surgeon must consider the size of the tear and tissue quality as well as repair tension when deciding when to begin phase 1 physical therapy. For larger or massive rotator cuff tears, tears under more tension, or individuals with other risk factors for poor healing, patients may be immobilized for up to 6 weeks without starting any therapy or motion. For patients who are immobilized for 6 weeks before initiating any type of therapy, phase 1 can be condensed into 2 weeks after initiation, and then phase 2 begins.

Phase 2

In phase 2 of rehabilitation, the general goals are to gradually restore range of motion and to initiate active muscle contractions with a focus on regaining proper scapula-humeral rhythm. Training in joint proprioception is begun during this phase, and a home exercise program should continue to be emphasized. This phase of rehabilitation should occur during weeks 6 through 12.

Range of motion should be progressed gradually as tolerated. At this stage, there are no restrictions on flexion, elevation, or internal and external rotation in the scapular plane. Exercises from phase 1 should be continued into phase 2, including active-assisted range of motion with a pulley or cane. Internal rotation stretching using a towel should be initiated if needed, as should posterior capsule stretching. Glenohumeral joint mobilizations should be continued, emphasizing posterior and inferior glides. Therapist-directed manual stretching should be performed after mobilizations. The patient should aim to achieve full range of motion by 10 to 12 weeks postoperatively.

Strengthening should be progressed during this phase of rehabilitation. Supine active range of motion may be initiated with no resistance. This may be progressed to partial sitting, sidelying, and standing over time. Internal and external rotation exercises using a Theraband band may also be initiated. A towel roll should be placed between the upper arm and torso, and the patient can side step while holding neutral internal and external rotation for isometric resistance. Biceps and triceps exercises may progress using a Theraband.

Therapeutic exercises may be begun during this phase, including flexion, scaption, empty can, and deceleration. Rhythmic stab exercise may progress as tolerated from supine, sidelying, partial sitting, to standing. Scapular strengthening should also be emphasized, including Theraband band-assisted seated rows, shrugs, and punches. Starting at week 8, 2-handed plyometrics may be initiated if the patient is able. These include ball toss with chest pass, overhead pass, and diagonals. Starting at week 10, isokinetic testing for internal and external rotation may be initiated. This should begin in neutral position, then may progress to the 90/90 position in the scapular plane. The goal of the isokinetic testing is for 80% strength compared with the contralateral side.

Proprioceptive neuromuscular rehabilitation with manual resistance should be used during this phase.[16,17] The patient should continue to use heat before therapy session and ice afterward and when needed. Acupuncture and transcutaneous electical nerve stimulation (TENS) stimulation may be used to assist with pain control during rehabilitation. Although these modalities have been shown not to influence patient outcomes at 6 months, both modalities may help patients with pain at rest.[17]

Phase 3

In phase 3 of rehabilitation, the main goals are to restore full active range of motion, progress strengthening and scapular stabilization exercises, and initiate more functional drills into the rehabilitation program. This phase should occur during weeks 12 through 14. Although tendon to bone healing begins earlier, organization of collagen fibrils does not begin until 8 weeks following repair, and Sharpey fibers do not form in significant amounts until 12 weeks following repair.[18] Due to these tendon to bone healing considerations, strengthening is not begun until at least 12 weeks after repair at the beginning of phase 3.[19]

Range of motion exercises should focus on achieving and maintaining a full range of motion. Therapist-directed mobilizations may be more aggressive if needed.

Strengthening should focus on hypertrophy and strengthening of the rotator cuff muscles. Lower intensities are used to prevent recruitment from the larger surrounding muscles. Hypertrophy is emphasized initially through a higher volume of repetitions. Following hypertrophy, strengthening can be initiated by increasing intensities and weight while lowering repetitions.

Patients may continue with the previously described Theraband exercises while increasing intensity, sets, and repetitions as able. They should continue with their therapeutic exercises, increasing sets and repetitions, with intensity up to 7 lbs maximum. A push-up progression may be initiated at this point, from wall, table or counter, knees, to regular push-up. Theraband band external rotation exercises in the 90/90 position should also be initiated with both slow and fast repetitions. Prone therapeutic exercises including scaption at 130° with the thumb up, horizontal abduction with the thumb up, extension with the palm down, and external rotation may also be initiated.

Phase 4

In the final phase of rehabilitation, the main goals are to build full functional strength and implement functional or sport-specific training. It is also important to establish a progressive gym program for continued strengthening and endurance training. This phase extends from week 14 to week 24, although the duration of outpatient physical therapy rather than a home or gym-directed program can vary based on patient needs and level of function.

Range of motion exercises should be continued as needed to maintain normal range. The patient may progress to one-handed plyometric exercises including ball toss and ball on the wall exercises. They may also progress to eccentric rotator cuff strengthening using deceleration plyo ball throws and Therabands. Large muscle exercises may be included, including shoulder press, latissimus pull downs, and bench press, provided that the elbow does not extend past the plane of the thorax.

SUMMARY

Rehabilitation following a rotator cuff repair is an important factor for achieving satisfactory patient outcomes. The rehabilitation should be tailored to an individual patient's needs and should advance through stages based on patient progression. Rehabilitation is often done under the direction of a physical therapist and can be divided into 4 phases during a 6-month period.

The goals of therapy are to protect the tendon repair and prevent injury to the repair while preventing stiffness and restoring strength and function to provide a good outcome for the patient. Consistent communication between the patient, therapist, and surgeon is paramount for a good result. The ability to create a patient-specific program will provide these complex patients an opportunity for improved function and pain relief.

CLINICS CARE POINTS

- Rehabilitation following rotator cuff repair must allow for the restoration of motion and strength while also protecting the repair and allowing tendon bone healing.
- Rehabilitation programs should be tailored to individual patient/host factors, tear characteristics, and their repair integrity/quality.
- Close communication with physical/occupational therapists can improve patient outcomes.

DISCLOSURE

A.M. Murthi disclosures: Royalties-Depuy Inc, Globus Medical, Ignite Orthopaedics; Consulting-Depuy, Zimmer Biomet, vTail, WorkRehabSolution, Aevumed.

REFERENCES

1. Fucentese SF, von Roll AL, Pfirrmann CW, et al. Evolution of nonoperatively treated symptomatic isolated full-thickness supraspinatus tears. J Bone Joint Surg Am 2012;94(9):801–8.
2. Lee BG, Cho NS, Rhee YG. Effect of two rehabilitation protocols on range of motion and healing rates after arthroscopic rotator cuff repair: aggressive versus limited early passive exercises. Arthroscopy 2012;28(1):34–42.
3. Chung SW, Huong CB, Kim SH, et al. Shoulder stiffness after rotator cuff repair: risk factors and influence on outcome. Arthroscopy 2013;29(2):290–300.
4. Galatz LM, Ball CM, Teefey SA, et al. The outcome and repair integrity of completely arthroscopically repaired large and massive rotator cuff tears. J Bone Joint Surg Am 2004;86(2):219–24.
5. Parsons BO, Gruson KI, Chen DD, et al. Does slower rehabilitation after arthroscopic rotator cuff repair lead to long-term stiffness? J Shoulder Elbow Surg 2010;19(7):1034–9.
6. Ross D, Maerz T, Lynch J, et al. Rehabilitation following arthroscopic rotator cuff repair: a review of current literature. J Am Acad Orthop Surg 2014;22(1):1–9.
7. Thigpen CA, Shaffer MA, Gaunt BW, et al. The American Society of Shoulder and Elbow Therapists' consensus statement on rehabilitation following arthroscopic rotator cuff repair. J Shoulder Elbow Surg 2016;25(4):521–35.
8. Gasbarro G, Ye J, Newsome H, et al. Morphologic risk factors in predicting symptomatic structural failure of arthroscopic rotator cuff repairs: tear size, location, and atrophy matter. Arthroscopy 2016;32(10):1947–52.
9. Kim IB, Jung DW. A rotator cuff tear concomitant with shoulder stiffness is associated with a lower retear rate after 1-stage arthroscopic surgery. Am J Sports Med 2018;46(8):1909–18.
10. Nho SJ, Brown BS, Lyman S, et al. Prospective analysis of arthroscopic rotator cuff repair: prognostic factors affecting clinical and ultrasound outcome. J Shoulder Elbow Surg 2009;18(1):13–20.
11. Jensen AR, Taylor AJ, Sanchez-Sotelo J. Factors influencing the reparability and healing rates of rotator cuff tears. Curr Rev Musculoskelet Med 2020;13(5):572–83.
12. Karppi P, Ryosa A, Kukkonen J, et al. Effectiveness of supervised physiotherapy after arthroscopic rotator cuff reconstruction: a randomized controlled trial. J Shoulder Elbow Surg 2020;29(9):1765–74.
13. Brennan GP, Parent EC, Cleland JA. Description of clinical outcomes and postoperative utilization of physical therapy services within 4 categories of shoulder surgery. J Orthop Sports Phys Ther 2010;40(1):20–9.
14. Tirefort J, Schwitzguebel AJ, Collin P, et al. Postoperative mobilization after superior rotator cuff repair: sling versus no sling: a randomized prospective study. J Bone Joint Surg Am 2019;101(6):494–503.
15. Mazzocca AD, Arciero RA, Shea KP, et al. The effect of early range of motion on quality of life, clinical outcome, and repair integrity after arthroscopic rotator cuff repair. Arthroscopy 2017;33(6):1138–48.

16. van der Meijden OA, Westgard P, Chandler Z, et al. Rehabilitation after arthroscopic rotator cuff repair: current concepts review and evidence-based guidelines. Int J Sports Phys Ther 2012;7(2):197–218.

17. Razavi M, Jansen GB. Effects of acupuncture and placebo TENS in addition to exercise in treatment of rotator cuff tendinitis. Clin Rehabil 2004;18(8):872–8.

18. Sonnabend DH, Howlett CR, Young AA. Histological evaluation of repair of the rotator cuff in a primate model. J Bone Joint Surg Br 2010;92(4):586–94.

19. Favard L, Bacle G, Berhouet J. Rotator cuff repair. Joint Bone Spine 2007;74(6): 551–7.

Nonoperative Treatment of the Biceps-Labral Complex

Suleiman Y. Sudah, MD[a,1], Mariano E. Menendez, MD[b], Grant E. Garrigues, MD[c,*]

KEYWORDS

• Biceps-labral complex • Long head of the biceps tendon • Labrum • Nonoperative

KEY POINTS

• Biceps-labral complex injuries are widely recognized as a source of anterior shoulder pain and dysfunction.
• Several studies have shown that relatively good outcomes—even in overhead athletes—may be achieved with nonoperative management.
• Nonsteroidal anti-inflammatory drugs, glucocorticoid injections, and physical therapy regimens focused on restoring muscle strength, endurance, neuromuscular control, and normal scapulothoracic/glenohumeral motion should be exhausted before considering operative intervention.

INTRODUCTION

Injuries to the long head of the biceps tendon (LHBT) and superior glenoid labrum are widely recognized as a source of anterior shoulder pain and dysfunction,[1–3] particularly in athletic and working individuals.[2] Although lesions to the LHBT and superior labrum have been traditionally viewed as separate entities, current literature has underscored the importance of viewing the biceps-labral complex (BLC) as an interdependent functional unit.[4,5] According to a large retrospective database study, the presence of concomitant biceps tendinitis or LHBT tear significantly increases the odds of superior labral anterior and posterior (SLAP) repair failure.[6] In fact, several studies have shown that SLAP tears can be successfully treated with biceps tenotomy or tenodesis in the absence of primary SLAP repair.[7–10]

However, surgical outcomes are mixed and a consensus regarding the optimal surgical management strategy for BLC injuries has not been reached.[11,12] Recently,

[a] Department of Orthopedics, Monmouth Medical Center, 300 2nd Avenue, Long Branch, NJ 07740, USA; [b] Oregon Shoulder Institute at Southern Oregon Orthopedics, 2780 East Barnett Road, 200, Medford, OR 97504, USA; [c] Department of Orthopaedic Surgery, Rush University Medical Center, Midwest Orthopaedics at Rush, 1611 West Harrison Street, Orthopedic Building, Suite 400, Chicago, IL 60612, USA
[1] Present address: 19 Clover Place, Franklin Park, NJ 08823.
* Corresponding author.
E-mail address: grant.garrigues@rushortho.com

Phys Med Rehabil Clin N Am 34 (2023) 365–375
https://doi.org/10.1016/j.pmr.2022.12.004
1047-9651/23/© 2022 Elsevier Inc. All rights reserved.

several studies have shown that relatively good outcomes—even in overhead athletes—may be achieved with nonoperative management.[13–17] Herein, we review the anatomy, pathogenesis, diagnosis, and outcomes of nonoperative treatment of BLC injuries.

Anatomy and Pathogenesis

The BLC is divided into three clinically relevant zones: inside, junction, and bicipital tunnel.[5] The inside zone includes the biceps anchor, which refers to the attachment of the LHBT onto the superior glenoid labrum and supraglenoid tubercle.[5] The attachment site of the LHBT on the superior labrum is variable, but most commonly has equal anterior and posterior attachment.[18] Injuries within this zone include SLAP tears and entrapment of the LHBT within the glenohumeral joint.[19] The junction includes the intra-articular portion of the proximal LHBT and its stabilizing pulley, which can be viewed during shoulder arthroscopy.[5] Junctional lesions include subscapularis tears with resulting LHBT instability and pulley lesions.[19] The bicipital tunnel includes the extra-articular portion of the LHBT from the articular margin to the subpectoral region.[5] This region is further subdivided into three anatomically distinct zones.[20] The first includes the bony groove, which extends from the articular margin to the distal margin of the subscapularis muscle (DMSS). The second zone extends from the DMSS to the proximal portion of the pectoralis major tendon. The third zone includes the subpectoralis region. The LHBT is roughly 9 cm in length from its origin to the musculotendinous junction.[21] It originates from the supraglenoid tubercle and labrum and passes posterior to the coracohumeral ligament (CHL) and inferior to the transverse humeral ligament.[22] A soft tissue sling created from fibers of the CHL and superior glenohumeral ligament (SGHL) acts to stabilize the tendon at the lateral apex of the rotator interval.

Lesions of the BLC are similarly classified into three categories: inflammatory (tendinitis), instability, and traumatic.[23] These injuries are often associated with a variety of other shoulder pathologies,[24] which include symptomatic tears of the rotator cuff,[25,26] coracohumeral and/or superior glenohumeral complex,[27,28] and glenohumeral osteoarthritis.[27] Between 45% and 82% of patients with symptomatic rotator cuff tears are found to have LHBT pathology.[29]

Primary biceps tendonitis is rare with incidence ranging from 0% to 5%.[30] Secondary causes are more common and mostly include impingement,[31] mechanical wear,[32] or inflammation of the glenohumeral joint.[22] Instability of the LHBT results from disruption of the soft tissue pulley system,[29] which occurs following injury to the CHL or SGHL, subscapularis tendon, or lesser tuberosity.[21,33] Primary traumatic rupture of the tendon is rare, with incidence ranging from 2% to 6%.[21] More commonly, rupture occurs as a consequence of chronic tendinopathy in the setting of rotator cuff tears.[34]

Several mechanisms for BLC injury in athletes have been described.[4] Andrews and colleagues[35] proposed that most tears of the glenoid labrum in throwing athletes occur at the anterosuperior portion and result from traction of the biceps tendon. In an electromyographic analysis of muscle activation in throwing athletes, increased activity of the biceps brachii was found in those with anterior glenohumeral instability.[36] This suggests that compensation of the biceps may lead to increased rates of SLAP tears in this population. Fleisig and colleagues[37] used high-speed motion analysis to study the implications of shoulder and elbow kinetics on injury mechanisms. It was suggested that grinding forces of the glenohumeral joint and tension of the biceps tendon due to elbow flexion torque and shoulder compressive force may contribute to anterior labrum and anterosuperior labrum tears, respectively. Burkhart and Morgan[38] described a "peel back" mechanism of labral injury resulting from torsional forces imposed by the LHBT that occur during repetitive overhead motion. Walch and colleagues[39] described the internal impingement theory, where the underside of the posterosuperior rotator cuff impinges on the posterosuperior labrum in 90° of abduction and 90° of external rotation. Repeated contact between the rotator cuff and labrum during overhead activity is a proposed mechanism of partial-thickness rotator cuff tears and SLAP lesions in throwers.[40]

DIAGNOSIS
History

Patients with BLC injuries report anterior shoulder pain that migrates into the anterior biceps; this pain is often exacerbated with elbow flexion and overhead activity.[27] In throwing athletes, anterior shoulder pain of the dominant arm with gradual loss of function and decreasing ball velocity should raise suspicion for injury to the BLC.[22,41] However, these symptoms are common to many shoulder pathologies—such partial-thickness rotator cuff tears, capsulolabral injuries, and internal impingement—which often coexist in athletes.[42] Patients may describe mechanical symptoms such as clicking or popping resulting from catching of the tendon in the anterior shoulder. These symptoms occur during the late cocking phase in throwers and during the serve in volleyball and tennis players.[22,43,44] Those with tendon rupture may exhibit the classic Popeye deformity with ecchymosis of the anterior arm and complaints of muscle cramping.[3]

Physical Examination

The physical examination is critical in the diagnosis of biceps and superior labral pathology. Glenohumeral and scapulothoracic motion should be evaluated bilaterally in the supine position, particularly in overhead athletes, as deficits in internal rotation and scapular motion are often present.[45] Pain with direct palpation over the bicipital groove located 7 cm distal to the acromion with the arm internally rotated 10° is the most common site of pain in those with LHBT pathology.[3,46] Evaluating strength of the rotator cuff muscles can help to diagnose potential rotator cuff tears. Assessment of subscapularis function is of particular importance in those with suspected biceps tendon instability.[47] In addition, shoulder stability tests should be performed as anterior capsulolabral injuries with SLAP tears are not uncommon.[48]

A variety of provocative tests have been described to aid in the diagnosis of BLC injuries. Among these are the O'Brien active compression, the modified O'Brien active compression, crank, Speed, anterior slide, Yergason, and dynamic labral shear tests.[49–55] A summary of these tests and their diagnostic capabilities has been previously published.[48,56] Most are associated with poor specificity and sensitivity (**Table 1**) and yield inconsistent diagnostic values when used alone or in combination.[49,51,57,58]

Imaging

Initial evaluation should include a complete radiographic shoulder series, including true anteroposterior, lateral, and axillary views.[48] Although no pathognomonic radiographic findings exist for BLC lesions, these studies help to identify the presence of coexisting bony lesions.[48] A recent systematic review and meta-analysis compared the diagnostic accuracy of magnetic resonance arthrography (MRA) and MRI for the diagnosis of SLAP tears.[59] MRA was found to have higher sensitivity (80.4% versus 63%) and specificity (90.7% versus 87%) compared with MRI. The utility of MRI to diagnose LHBT pathology is less predictable and varies by tendon location.[60,61] Taylor and colleagues[61] reported a sensitivity of 43.3% and 50.4% and specificity of 55.6%

Table 1
Provocative tests for the diagnosis of superior labral anterior and posterior tears with reported diagnostic performance[a]

Test	Sensitivity, %	Specificity, %	PPV, %	NPV, %
O'Brien active compression test	47 to 100	11.1 to 98.5	10 to 94.6	14.3 to 100
Anterior slide test	8 to 78.4	81.5 to 91.5	5 to 66.7	67.6 to 90
Bicep load test I	90.9	96.9	83	98
Bicep load test II	89.7	96.9	92.1	95.5
Crank test	12.5 to 91	56 to 100	41 to 100	29 to 90
Pain provocation test	15 to 100	90 to 90.2	40 to 95	70.9 to 100
Resisted supination external rotation test	82.8	81.8	92.3	64.3
Rotation compression test	24 to 25	76 to 100	9 to 100	58 to 90
Forced abduction test	67	67	62	71
Yergason test	43	79	60	65
Speed test	32	75	50	58

Abbreviations: NPV, negative predictive value; PPV, positive predictive value.
[a] Data reported as a range or single value.
Adapted from Knesek M, Skendzel JG, Dines JS, Altchek DW, Allen AA, Bedi A. Diagnosis and management of superior labral anterior posterior tears in throwing athletes. Am J Sports Med. Feb 2013;41(2):444-60. https://doi.org/10.1177/0363546512466067.

and 61.4% when MRI is used for the diagnosis of junctional and bicipital tunnel lesions, respectively. MRI can also be associated with clinically false-positive findings. In a study of 20 asymptomatic overhead athletes,[62] partial- or full-thickness rotator cuff tears were diagnosed in 8 (40%) of the dominant shoulders compared with none in the nondominant shoulder. The authors concluded that MRI alone should not be used as a determinant for operative intervention, which highlights the importance of a detailed clinical history and physical examination in the evaluation of BLC injuries.

Clinical Relevance of Imaging Findings

Substantial interobserver variability in the diagnosis of SLAP tears was previously shown.[63] Seventy-three expert surgeons were tasked with reviewing 22 arthroscopic video vignettes to classify SLAP lesions and provide a treatment recommendation for each vignette. Only 68% of surgeons correctly diagnosed the non-pathologic shoulders, with 29% of surgeons recommending either arthroscopic debridement or labral repair for incorrectly diagnosed type I and II SLAP tears.

There are several normal variants of labral morphology that have been described in the anterior and superior glenoid region. These variants make the diagnosis of BLC injuries difficult as they are likely to occur in similar locations. MRI assessment of 52 asymptomatic shoulders showed extensive variability in the morphology of the anterior and posterior parts of the labra, respectively: triangular (45%, 73%), round (19%, 12%), cleaved (15%, 0%), notched (8%, 0%), flat (7%, 6%), and absent (6%, 8%).[64]

A sublabral foramen (Buford complex) is a normal labral variant that is commonly confused with an SLAP tear or anterior labral tear on MRI.[65,66] It is formed by a focal detachment of the anterosuperior labrum from the glenoid and may be present in up to 20% of shoulder MRIs.[66,67] Differentiating between normal variants and SLAP tears is important to guide treatment decisions. This is particularly relevant for the elderly population who have worse outcomes after SLAP repair[68] and a high prevalence of normal labral variants.[69] Thus, it is critical for shoulder surgeons to determine which SLAP tears are symptomatic and which are asymptomatic or normal variants.

Nonoperative Treatment

Initial treatment strategies for BLC injuries should focus on nonoperative intervention. Management begins with activity modification and nonsteroidal anti-inflammatory (NSAIDs) medications for pain control, with progression to anesthetic and corticosteroid injections in refractory cases.[70] Peritendinous or bicipital sheath injections may have diagnostic and therapeutic value.[71–74] However, there is a risk of tendon rupture with steroid injections[75] and their efficacy in treating chronic injuries has been questioned.[76] Although other injection-based therapies such as prolotherapy, platelet-rich plasma, and stem cells have emerged,[77,78] there is little data to support their use for BLC injuries. NSAIDs and/or intra-articular injections should be used as an adjunct to a physical therapy program.[79] The goals of physical therapy are to restore muscle strength, endurance, neuromuscular control, and normal scapulothoracic/glenohumeral motion. For throwing athletes the goals are to restore total arc of motion and optimize pitching motion to avoid internal impingement positions. It is recommended that operative intervention be considered in those who fail to improve with physical therapy after 3 to 6 months,[79] which is characterized by the inability to regain painless range of motion, rotator cuff strength, or return to prior activity level.[13,15]

Outcomes of Nonoperative Treatment

Most of the literature on BLC disease has focused on surgical outcomes, with few studies evaluating the success of nonsurgical management.[13–17] Edwards and colleagues[13] were among the first to evaluate outcomes of conservatively managed SLAP tears. Validated, patient-derived outcome instruments were mailed to 371 patients with this diagnosis. Of the 39 respondents who met the inclusion criteria, 19 were successfully treated nonoperatively and 20 elected to undergo arthroscopic surgery. The average age of those in the nonoperative group was 34 years and all identified as athletes at the recreational or competitive level. At an average follow-up of 3.1 years, significant improvements in function (American Shoulder and Elbow Score, ASES, 30.8–45, $P < .001$; Simple Shoulder Test, SST, 8.3–11, $P = .02$), pain (Visual Analog Pain Scale, VAS, 4.5–2.1, $P = .043$), and quality of life (EuroQol 0.76–0.89, $P = .009$) were found compared with pre-treatment levels. Comparable functional improvements have been reported in those undergoing SLAP repair with similar follow-up periods.[80,81] In addition, all but two patients returned to sports within 6 months, with 71% achieving pre-participation levels. Although performance was lower in overhead athletes (66.6% returning to or exceeding pre-injury levels), this finding is generally consistent in those who undergo surgery.[82,83] Similar findings were reported in a slightly larger study of 63 patients who initially underwent nonoperative treatment for isolated type II SLAP tears. At an average follow-up of 21 months, 71.4% (45/63) achieved significant improvements in function (ASES, 54.2–86.4) and pain (VAS 4.6–1.7; $P < .05$) without surgery. Eighteen (28.5%) patients comprised the failure group, which included patients who underwent arthroscopic surgery or had <20-point improvement in ASES score and inability to return to activities. It was found that patients engaged in overhead activity were less likely to succeed with nonoperative management. However, surgical outcomes in overhead athletes are inconsistent,[81] which makes it difficult to ascertain whether conversion to surgery would be useful.

Fedoriw[15] et al assessed return to play (RTP) and return to prior performance (RPP) after surgical and nonsurgical treatment of SLAP tears in 68 professional baseball players. All players had failed an initial attempt at rehabilitation before presentation. A second attempt at physical therapy was required before surgical consultation. This included a supervised regimen that focused on correcting scapular dyskinesia and posterior capsular contracture with glenohumeral internal rotation deficit (GIRD), followed by pain-free return to motion. The success rate for those undergoing nonoperative intervention was 40% (18/45) for pitchers and 39% (9/23) for position players. For those treated nonoperatively, RTP was 85.7% (18/21) for pitchers and 90% (9/10) for position players and the RPP was 22% (10/45) and 26% (6/23), respectively. Although the RPP seems low, these rates are similar to what was reported for surgically-treated players. RTP for less than one season, RTP with a decline in performance statistics, or RTP to a less competitive league were factors that precluded an RPP. Although the authors acknowledge the stringency of these measures, they advocate the use of RPP in place of traditionally reported RTP rates.[84,85] It was ultimately concluded that nonsurgical treatment should be considered in professional baseball pitchers with SLAP tears because it can be successful and because surgery may be unable to considerably improve performance in those who fail conservative measures.

Steinmetz and colleagues[14] systematically reviewed outcomes following nonsurgical management of SLAP tears. A total of five articles including 244 athletes with a mean age from 20.3 to 38 years were analyzed. Overall, 53.7% of athletes returned to play and 42.6% returned to prior performance. Interestingly, these rates increased to 78% and 72%, respectively, for those who completed their rehabilitation programs. These data support the relatively positive results of nonoperatively managed SLAP tears, particularly in those who are able to complete their physical therapy protocol before returning to play. However, this review was limited by the retrospective nature and heterogeneity of included studies, which include differences in activity levels (athletes versus non-athletes), the definitions of athletic prowess ("elite" or "high level"), sport type, and rehabilitation protocols.

SUMMARY

The LHBT and superior labrum should be evaluated as an interdependent functional unit. BLC injuries are difficult to diagnose and often associated with other shoulder pathologies. A focused patient history and physical examination including multiple provocative tests should be performed alongside advanced imaging studies. Significant improvements in pain, functional outcomes and quality of life are achieved in most patients treated nonoperatively. Nonoperative treatment modalities including NSAIDs, glucocorticoid injections, throwing evaluation for pitching optimization, and physical therapy should be exhausted before considering operative intervention. Although outcomes are less consistent for overhead athletes, RTP and prior performance appear comparable among those treated with and without surgery. High-quality, prospective study designs and uniformity in nonoperative treatment protocols, particularly among overhead athletes, are needed to further understand the role of conservatively managed BLC injuries.

CLINICS CARE POINTS

- The LHBT and superior labrum should be evaluated as an interdependent functional unit.
- A focused patient history and physical examination including multiple provocative tests should be performed alongside advanced imaging studies.

- Nonoperative treatment modalities including NSAIDs, glucocorticoid injections, throwing evaluation for pitching optimization, and physical therapy should be exhausted before considering operative intervention.

- Significant improvements in pain, functional outcomes and quality of life are achieved in most patients treated nonoperatively.

DISCLOSURE

S.Y. Sudah has no disclosures. M.E. Menendez is a consultant for Arthrex Inc. G.E. Garriagues has the following disclosures: Additive Orthopedics: Paid consultant American Shoulder and Elbow Surgeons: Board or committee member Arthrex, Inc: Other financial or material support Arthroscopy Association of North America: Board or committee member CultivateMD: Stock or stock Options DJ Orthopedics: IP royalties; Other financial or material support; Paid consultant; Paid presenter or speaker Genesys: Stock or stock Options Journal of Shoulder and Elbow Surgery: Editorial or governing board Mitek: Paid consultant Patient IQ: Stock or stock Options ROM 3: Stock or stock Options SouthTech: Other financial or material support Techniques in Orthopedics: Editorial or governing board Tornier: IP royalties; Paid consultant; Paid presenter or speaker.

REFERENCES

1. Lalehzarian SP, Agarwalla A, Liu JN. Management of proximal biceps tendon pathology. World J Orthop 2022;13(1):36–57.
2. Krupp RJ, Kevern MA, Gaines MD, et al. Long head of the biceps tendon pain: differential diagnosis and treatment. J Orthop Sports Phys Ther 2009;39(2): 55–70.
3. Frank RM, Cotter EJ, Strauss EJ, et al. Management of Biceps Tendon Pathology: From the Glenoid to the Radial Tuberosity. Instr Course Lect 2018;67:439–52.
4. Calcei JG, Boddapati V, Altchek DW, et al. Diagnosis and Treatment of Injuries to the Biceps and Superior Labral Complex in Overhead Athletes. Curr Rev Musculoskelet Med 2018;11(1):63–71.
5. Taylor SA, O'Brien SJ. Clinically Relevant Anatomy and Biomechanics of the Proximal Biceps. Clin Sports Med 2016;35(1):1–18.
6. Taylor SA, Degen RM, White AE, et al. Risk factors for revision surgery after superior labral anterior-posterior repair: a national perspective. Am J Sports Med 2017;45(7):1640–4.
7. Patterson BM, Creighton RA, Spang JT, et al. Surgical Trends in the Treatment of Superior Labrum Anterior and Posterior Lesions of the Shoulder: Analysis of Data From the American Board of Orthopaedic Surgery Certification Examination Database. Am J Sports Med 2014;42(8):1904–10.
8. Boileau P, Parratte S, Chuinard C, et al. Arthroscopic treatment of isolated type II SLAP lesions: biceps tenodesis as an alternative to reinsertion. Am J Sports Med 2009;37(5):929–36.
9. Ek ET, Shi LL, Tompson JD, et al. Surgical treatment of isolated type II superior labrum anterior-posterior (SLAP) lesions: repair versus biceps tenodesis. J Shoulder Elbow Surg 2014;23(7):1059–65.
10. Denard PJ, Ladermann A, Parsley BK, et al. Arthroscopic biceps tenodesis compared with repair of isolated type II SLAP lesions in patients older than 35 years. Orthopedics 2014;37(3):e292–7.

11. Mazzocca AD, Cote MP, Arciero CL, et al. Clinical outcomes after subpectoral biceps tenodesis with an interference screw. Am J Sports Med 2008;36(10):1922–9.

12. Boileau P, Baque F, Valerio L, et al. Isolated arthroscopic biceps tenotomy or tenodesis improves symptoms in patients with massive irreparable rotator cuff tears. J Bone Joint Surg Am 2007;89(4):747–57.

13. Edwards SL, Lee JA, Bell JE, et al. Nonoperative treatment of superior labrum anterior posterior tears: improvements in pain, function, and quality of life. Am J Sports Med 2010;38(7):1456–61.

14. Steinmetz RG, Guth JJ, Matava MJ, et al. Return to play following nonsurgical management of superior labrum anterior-posterior tears: a systematic review. J Shoulder Elbow Surg 2022;31(6):1323–33.

15. Fedoriw WW, Ramkumar P, McCulloch PC, et al. Return to play after treatment of superior labral tears in professional baseball players. Am J Sports Med 2014;42(5):1155–60.

16. Jang SH, Seo JG, Jang HS, et al. Predictive factors associated with failure of nonoperative treatment of superior labrum anterior-posterior tears. J Shoulder Elbow Surg 2016;25(3):428–34.

17. Hashiguchi H, Iwashita S, Yoneda M, et al. Factors influencing outcomes of nonsurgical treatment for baseball players with SLAP lesion. Asia Pac J Sports Med Arthrosc Rehabil Technol 2018;14:6–9.

18. Vangsness CT Jr, Jorgenson SS, Watson T, et al. The origin of the long head of the biceps from the scapula and glenoid labrum. An anatomical study of 100 shoulders. J Bone Joint Surg Br 1994;76(6):951–4.

19. Wilk KE, Hooks TR. The Painful Long Head of the Biceps Brachii: Nonoperative Treatment Approaches. Clin Sports Med 2016;35(1):75–92.

20. Taylor SA, Fabricant PD, Bansal M, et al. The anatomy and histology of the bicipital tunnel of the shoulder. J Shoulder Elbow Surg 2015;24(4):511–9.

21. Habermeyer P, Magosch P, Pritsch M, et al. Anterosuperior impingement of the shoulder as a result of pulley lesions: a prospective arthroscopic study. J Shoulder Elbow Surg 2004;13(1):5–12.

22. Barber A, Field LD, Ryu R. Biceps tendon and superior labrum injuries: decision-marking. J Bone Joint Surg Am 2007;89(8):1844–55.

23. Schickendantz M, King D. Nonoperative Management (Including Ultrasound-Guided Injections) of Proximal Biceps Disorders. Clin Sports Med 2016;35(1):57–73.

24. Hsu SH, Miller SL, Curtis AS. Long head of biceps tendon pathology: management alternatives. Clin Sports Med 2008;27(4):747–62.

25. Vestermark GL, Van Doren BA, Connor PM, et al. The prevalence of rotator cuff pathology in the setting of acute proximal biceps tendon rupture. J Shoulder Elbow Surg 2018;27(7):1258–62.

26. Murthi AM, Vosburgh CL, Neviaser TJ. The incidence of pathologic changes of the long head of the biceps tendon. J Shoulder Elbow Surg 2000;9(5):382–5.

27. Frank RM, Cotter EJ, Strauss EJ, et al. Management of Biceps Tendon Pathology: From the Glenoid to the Radial Tuberosity. J Am Acad Orthop Surg 2018;26(4):e77–89.

28. Patel KV, Bravman J, Vidal A, et al. Biceps Tenotomy Versus Tenodesis. Clin Sports Med 2016;35(1):93–111.

29. Lafosse L, Reiland Y, Baier GP, et al. Anterior and posterior instability of the long head of the biceps tendon in rotator cuff tears: a new classification based on arthroscopic observations. Arthroscopy 2007;23(1):73–80.

30. Friedman DJ, Dunn JC, Higgins LD, et al. Proximal biceps tendon: injuries and management. Sports Med Arthrosc Rev 2008;16(3):162–9.
31. Slatis P, Aalto K. Medial dislocation of the tendon of the long head of the biceps brachii. Acta Orthop Scand 1979;50(1):73–7.
32. Neer CS 2nd. Anterior acromioplasty for the chronic impingement syndrome in the shoulder: a preliminary report. J Bone Joint Surg Am 1972;54(1):41–50.
33. Walch G, Nove-Josserand L, Boileau P, et al. Subluxations and dislocations of the tendon of the long head of the biceps. J Shoulder Elbow Surg 1998;7(2):100–8.
34. Packer NP, Calvert PT, Bayley JI, et al. Operative treatment of chronic ruptures of the rotator cuff of the shoulder. J Bone Joint Surg Br 1983;65(2):171–5.
35. Andrews JR, Carson WG Jr, McLeod WD. Glenoid labrum tears related to the long head of the biceps. Am J Sports Med 1985;13(5):337–41.
36. Jobe FW, Moynes DR, Tibone JE, et al. An EMG analysis of the shoulder in pitching. A second report. Am J Sports Med 1984;12(3):218–20.
37. Fleisig GS, Andrews JR, Dillman CJ, et al. Kinetics of baseball pitching with implications about injury mechanisms. Am J Sports Med 1995;23(2):233–9.
38. Burkhart SS, Morgan CD. The peel-back mechanism: its role in producing and extending posterior type II SLAP lesions and its effect on SLAP repair rehabilitation. Arthroscopy 1998;14(6):637–40.
39. Walch G, Liotard JP, Boileau P, et al. [Postero-superior glenoid impingement. Another impingement of the shoulder]. J Radiol 1993;74(1):47–50. Le conflit glenoidien postero-superieur. Un autre conflit de l'epaule.
40. Greiwe RM, Ahmad CS. Management of the throwing shoulder: cuff, labrum and internal impingement. Orthop Clin North Am 2010;41(3):309–23.
41. Bedi A, Allen AA. Superior labral lesions anterior to posterior-evaluation and arthroscopic management. Clin Sports Med 2008;27(4):607–30.
42. Angelo RL. The overhead athlete: how to examine, test, and treat shoulder injuries. Intra-articular pathology. Arthroscopy 2003;19(Suppl 1):47–50.
43. Keener JD, Brophy RH. Superior labral tears of the shoulder: pathogenesis, evaluation, and treatment. J Am Acad Orthop Surg 2009;17(10):627–37.
44. Dines JS, Bedi A, Williams PN, et al. Tennis injuries: epidemiology, pathophysiology, and treatment. J Am Acad Orthop Surg 2015;23(3):181–9.
45. Burkhart SS, Morgan CD, Kibler WB. The disabled throwing shoulder: spectrum of pathology Part III: The SICK scapula, scapular dyskinesis, the kinetic chain, and rehabilitation. Arthroscopy 2003;19(6):641–61.
46. Chalmers PN, Verma NN. Proximal Biceps in Overhead Athletes. Clin Sports Med 2016;35(1):163–79.
47. Hegedus EJ, Goode A, Campbell S, et al. Physical examination tests of the shoulder: a systematic review with meta-analysis of individual tests. Br J Sports Med 2008;42(2):80–92 ; discussion 92.
48. Knesek M, Skendzel JG, Dines JS, et al. Diagnosis and management of superior labral anterior posterior tears in throwing athletes. Am J Sports Med 2013;41(2):444–60.
49. Kim SH, Ha KI, Ahn JH, et al. Biceps load test II: A clinical test for SLAP lesions of the shoulder. Arthroscopy 2001;17(2):160–4.
50. McCaughey R, Green RA, Taylor NF. The anatomical basis of the resisted supination external rotation test for superior labral anterior to posterior lesions. Clin Anat 2009;22(6):665–70.
51. McFarland EG, Kim TK, Savino RM. Clinical assessment of three common tests for superior labral anterior-posterior lesions. Am J Sports Med 2002;30(6):810–5.

52. Schlechter JA, Summa S, Rubin BD. The passive distraction test: a new diagnostic aid for clinically significant superior labral pathology. Arthroscopy 2009; 25(12):1374–9.

53. Walsworth MK, Doukas WC, Murphy KP, et al. Reliability and diagnostic accuracy of history and physical examination for diagnosing glenoid labral tears. Am J Sports Med 2008;36(1):162–8.

54. Urch E, Taylor SA, Zitkovsky H, et al. A Modification of the Active Compression Test for the Shoulder Biceps-Labrum Complex. Arthrosc Tech 2017;6(3):e859–62.

55. O'Brien SJ, Pagnani MJ, Fealy S, et al. The active compression test: a new and effective test for diagnosing labral tears and acromioclavicular joint abnormality. Am J Sports Med 1998;26(5):610–3.

56. Holtby R, Razmjou H. Accuracy of the Speed's and Yergason's tests in detecting biceps pathology and SLAP lesions: comparison with arthroscopic findings. Arthroscopy 2004;20(3):231–6.

57. Cook C, Beaty S, Kissenberth MJ, et al. Diagnostic accuracy of five orthopedic clinical tests for diagnosis of superior labrum anterior posterior (SLAP) lesions. J Shoulder Elbow Surg 2012;21(1):13–22.

58. Meserve BB, Cleland JA, Boucher TR. A meta-analysis examining clinical test utility for assessing superior labral anterior posterior lesions. Am J Sports Med 2009; 37(11):2252–8.

59. Symanski JS, Subhas N, Babb J, et al. Diagnosis of Superior Labrum Anterior-to-Posterior Tears by Using MR Imaging and MR Arthrography: A Systematic Review and Meta-Analysis. Radiology 2017;285(1):101–13.

60. Taylor SA, Khair MM, Gulotta LV, et al. Diagnostic glenohumeral arthroscopy fails to fully evaluate the biceps-labral complex. Arthroscopy 2015;31(2):215–24.

61. Taylor SA, Newman AM, Nguyen J, et al. Magnetic Resonance Imaging Currently Fails to Fully Evaluate the Biceps-Labrum Complex and Bicipital Tunnel. Arthroscopy 2016;32(2):238–44.

62. Connor PM, Banks DM, Tyson AB, et al. Magnetic resonance imaging of the asymptomatic shoulder of overhead athletes: a 5-year follow-up study. Am J Sports Med 2003;31(5):724–7.

63. Gobezie R, Zurakowski D, Lavery K, et al. Analysis of interobserver and intraobserver variability in the diagnosis and treatment of SLAP tears using the Snyder classification. Am J Sports Med 2008;36(7):1373–9.

64. Neumann CH, Petersen SA, Jahnke AH. MR imaging of the labral-capsular complex: normal variations. AJR Am J Roentgenol 1991;157(5):1015–21.

65. Tuite MJ, Blankenbaker DG, Seifert M, et al. Sublabral foramen and buford complex: inferior extent of the unattached or absent labrum in 50 patients. Radiology 2002;223(1):137–42.

66. Dunham KS, Bencardino JT, Rokito AS. Anatomic variants and pitfalls of the labrum, glenoid cartilage, and glenohumeral ligaments. Magn Reson Imaging Clin N Am 2012;20(2):213–28, x.

67. Rao AG, Kim TK, Chronopoulos E, et al. Anatomical variants in the anterosuperior aspect of the glenoid labrum: a statistical analysis of seventy-three cases. J Bone Joint Surg Am 2003;85(4):653–9.

68. Erickson J, Lavery K, Monica J, et al. Surgical treatment of symptomatic superior labrum anterior-posterior tears in patients older than 40 years: a systematic review. Am J Sports Med 2015;43(5):1274–82.

69. Pappas ND, Hall DC, Lee DH. Prevalence of labral tears in the elderly. J Shoulder Elbow Surg 2013;22(6):e11–5.

70. Nho SJ, Strauss EJ, Lenart BA, et al. Long head of the biceps tendinopathy: diagnosis and management. J Am Acad Orthop Surg 2010;18(11):645–56.
71. Lenz R, Kieb M, Diehl P, et al. [Muscle, tendon and joint injections : What is the evidence?]. Orthopade 2016;45(5):459–68. Injektionen an Muskeln, Sehnen und Gelenken : Was ist die Evidenz?
72. Barile A, La Marra A, Arrigoni F, et al. Anaesthetics, steroids and platelet-rich plasma (PRP) in ultrasound-guided musculoskeletal procedures. Br J Radiol 2016;89(1065):20150355.
73. Stone TJ, Adler RS. Ultrasound-Guided Biceps Peritendinous Injections in the Absence of a Distended Tendon Sheath: A Novel Rotator Interval Approach. J Ultrasound Med 2015;34(12):2287–92.
74. Gofeld M, Hurdle MF, Agur A. Biceps tendon sheath injection: an anatomical conundrum. Pain Med 2019;20(1):138–42.
75. Andres BM, Murrell GA. Treatment of tendinopathy: what works, what does not, and what is on the horizon. Clin Orthop Relat Res 2008;466(7):1539–54.
76. Childress MA, Beutler A. Management of chronic tendon injuries. Am Fam Physician 2013;87(7):486–90.
77. Mautner K, Blazuk J. Where do injectable stem cell treatments apply in treatment of muscle, tendon, and ligament injuries? PM R 2015;7(4 Suppl):S33–40.
78. Finnoff JT, Fowler SP, Lai JK, et al. Treatment of chronic tendinopathy with ultrasound-guided needle tenotomy and platelet-rich plasma injection. PM R 2011;3(10):900–11.
79. Michener LA, Abrams JS, Bliven KCH, et al. National athletic trainers' association position statement: evaluation, management, and outcomes of and return-to- play criteria for overhead athletes with superior labral anterior-posterior injuries. J Athl Train 2018;53(3):209–29.
80. O'Brien SJ, Allen AA, Coleman SH, et al. The trans-rotator cuff approach to SLAP lesions: technical aspects for repair and a clinical follow-up of 31 patients at a minimum of 2 years. Arthroscopy 2002;18(4):372–7.
81. Cohen DB, Coleman S, Drakos MC, et al. Outcomes of isolated type II SLAP lesions treated with arthroscopic fixation using a bioabsorbable tack. Arthroscopy 2006;22(2):136–42.
82. Sciascia A, Myers N, Kibler WB, et al. Return to preinjury levels of participation after superior labral repair in overhead athletes: a systematic review. J Athl Train 2015;50(7):767–77.
83. Gorantla K, Gill C, Wright RW. The outcome of type II SLAP repair: a systematic review. Arthroscopy 2010;26(4):537–45.
84. Cerynik DL, Ewald TJ, Sastry A, et al. Outcomes of isolated glenoid labral injuries in professional baseball pitchers. Clin J Sport Med 2008;18(3):255–8.
85. Neri BR, ElAttrache NS, Owsley KC, et al. Outcome of type II superior labral anterior posterior repairs in elite overhead athletes: Effect of concomitant partial-thickness rotator cuff tears. Am J Sports Med 2011;39(1):114–20.

Postoperative Rehabilitation After Superior Labrum Anterior Posterior Repair

Alyssa D. Althoff, MD*, Colby Brunette, BS,
Stephen Brockmeier, MD

KEYWORDS

- Rehabilitation • SLAP repair • Postoperative

KEY POINTS

- Patients commonly return to preinjury levels of function following superior labrum anterior posterior repairs and extensive postoperative rehabilitation.
- Successful recovery requires an initial focus on minimizing stress on the repair, followed by a gradual increase in range of motion and strength.
- Return to play is based on severity of original injury, rate of rehabilitation, reestablishment of range of motion as well as consideration to sport-specific or activity-specific physical demands.

INTRODUCTION

Injuries to the superior labrum of the glenohumeral joint were originally described as a common shoulder pathologic condition in overhead athletes by Andrews and colleagues in 1985.[1] Snyder and colleagues[2] later popularized the moniker superior labrum anterior posterior (SLAP) tears and further classified the pathology in 1990, yet it remains an entity that is challenging to both diagnose and manage.

Epidemiology, Pathophysiology, and Pathoanatomy

SLAP tears account for 1% to 3% of all sports medicine referrals, and the incidence continues to increase.[3–5] Patients with SLAP tears are more commonly men (3:1) and in the 20 to 29-year-old or 40 to 49-year-old age groups.[5] Overhead athletes and those involved heavily in throwing are at greatest risk.[6,7] Injury to the superior labrum occurs in the setting of several identified mechanisms. Direct compression

Department of Orthopaedic Surgery, University of Virginia, 2280 Ivy Road, Charlottesville, VA, USA
* Corresponding author.
E-mail address: ada7dx@virginia.edu

Phys Med Rehabil Clin N Am 34 (2023) 377–392
https://doi.org/10.1016/j.pmr.2022.12.005
1047-9651/23/© 2022 Elsevier Inc. All rights reserved.

of the humeral head against glenoid occurs due to acute trauma, such as a fall on an outstretched or abducted arm, or during contact sports. Traction or pull injuries can cause avulsion of the biceps tendon, as can eccentric lengthening. Chronic use and degeneration can also be key contributors to subsequent injury.[7-10] Compression and shear forces occur in the case of repetitive overhead movement or throwing.

SLAP tears are classically categorized into 4 types (**Fig. 1**). In type I tears, the superior labrum is frayed but remains attached. Type II tears may include fraying and degeneration but is defined by a detachment of the superior biceps-labral complex from the glenoid fossa. Type III tears involve a bucket-handle tear of the labrum, with an intact biceps' tendon. Type IV tears have the same bucket handle tear as type III but involve a partial tear of the biceps' tendon.[2] Type II tears are the most common variant requiring clinical care and/or operative intervention and will be the subject of the majority of this article, as will type IV tears that involve repair of biceps tendon.[3,6,8,9,11-13] Several additional classification schemes exist that expand on Snyder's original description but are presently outside the scope of this article.[14-17]

DIAGNOSIS AND SURGICAL INTERVENTION
Diagnosis

Clinical diagnosis of SLAP tears has been historically difficult.[8,18] Symptoms of a SLAP tear overlap with a number of other shoulder injuries, and many patients may have concomitant pathology.[19] Diagnosis of a clinically relevant tear by a practicing physician involves a comprehensive history, physical examination, and advanced imaging review.

There is controversy as to whether any single physical examination maneuver has been shown to be both sensitive and specific for SLAP tears.[20,21] However, there are 5 highly sensitive tests that can aid in diagnosis—the active compression (O'Brien), biceps load II, dynamic labral shear (O'Driscoll), Speed test, and labral

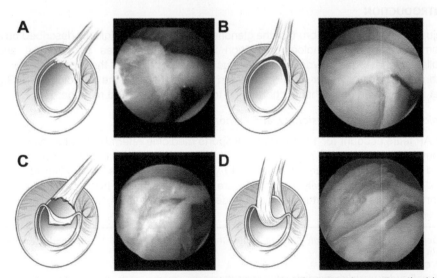

Fig. 1. The arthroscopic photo of the original SLAP tear classification scheme described by Snyder et al.[2] (A) Type I, (B) Type II, (C) Type II, and (D) Type IV. (*From* Werner BC, Brockmeier SF, Miller MD. Etiology, Diagnosis, and Management of Failed SLAP Repair. J Am Acad Orthop Surg. 2014;22(9):554-565. https://doi.org/10.5435/JAAOS-22-09-554.)

tension test.[22] Although physical examination is suggestive, subsequent pathology can be confirmed arthroscopically.

Range of motion, strengthen, and pain provocation maneuvers are recorded preoperatively and both the contralateral shoulder and the preoperative tests can be used to evaluate the patient's progress during postoperative rehabilitation.

Surgical Intervention

Surgical intervention, as decided on by the surgeon and patient, is guided by patient characteristics and presentation, examination, corresponding imaging evaluation, and arthroscopic visualization of the lesion. Type I tears may be addressed by debridement but do not necessitate repair. Degenerative type II tears commonly do not require repair, particularly when associated with additional pathologic condition but may be managed with debridement and/or biceps tenodesis. Type III tears may be managed with debridement, or debridement and repair. Finally, type IV tears may be addressed through debridement and biceps tenodesis, plus or minus primary labral repair. Primary repair is the treatment of choice for athletes and patients aged younger than 40 years.

Type II SLAP repairs have excellent clinical outcomes in terms of patient satisfaction, regain of function, and return to competitive play. Several studies have shown that greater than 80% of patients have "great" or "excellent" satisfaction rates.[9,11,23,24] Return to play rates have more variability, with a 2018 systemic review by Gorantla and colleagues[11] citing rates as high as 94%. Overhead throwers tend to have worse return to play returns compared with other athletes.[9,11,23,24] Similarly, acute traumatic injuries seem to have a better prognosis than chronic wear and tear.[9]

REHABILITATION
Overview

The current literature lacks high-quality empiric prospective trials evaluating the optimal postoperative rehabilitation protocol in this patient population.[8,25] In absence of such data, protocols such as the one listed in this article are based on an in-depth understanding of pathoanatomy, cadaveric studies, literature review, and experience with such injuries.

A general protocol that can be modified to meet the needs of individual patient goals is guided by the principle of gradual return to function. Postoperative rehabilitation varies based on the initial injury, extent of surgical repair, and the patient's functional goals. Throughout each phase, there are recommended limits to the degree of range of motion in various planes, reducing the stress on the repair in the early postoperative setting. As the repair heals, the focus transitions to strengthening and stability of the glenohumeral scapulothoracic articulations. In the later stages of rehabilitation, the emphasis shifts to improving and rebuilding preinjury levels of strength and conditioning. Patients finally progress to a continual maintenance phase, embedded in which is return to play.

Patient Evaluation

Evaluation during the rehabilitation process is a continuation of the initial patient evaluation. Important factors to consider are the patient's previous baseline function, the patient's goals for postrehab functional status, age, handedness, and extent of initial injury. An understanding of the surgical intervention performed, adjunct training may be required to maintain conditioning of the contralateral limb, core, and lower body.

Return to preinjury function will be based on subjective and objective measures including range of motion, strength, or ability. Contralateral limb measurements may

A

Restrictions
Shoulder sling x 6 weeks
Sleeping in sling x 3 weeks
No resisted active isolated biceps activity (elbow flexion or forearm supination x 6 weeks)
No active external shoulder rotation, extension, or abduction

Protocol
Hand gripping exercises
Passive and gentle active assisted ROM exercises
Codmans exercises
Flexion and scaption to 90^0
Eternal rotation (ER) to 30^0 x 4 weeks (passive)
Internal rotation (IR) to 45^0
Scapulothoracic AROM in all planes
Submaximal isometrics for shoulder musculature
Cryotherapy PRN

Weeks 3–4

Restrictions
Continue shoulder sling x 6 weeks
Discontinue sleeping in sling at end of 3 weeks
Continue no resisted active isolated biceps activity (elbow flexion or forearm supination x 6 weeks)
Continue no active ER, extension, or elevation

Protocol
Continue shoulder, elbow, and hand ROM (as above)
Advance IR to 60^0
Initiate scapulothoracic isometrics
Initiate proprioceptive training (rhythmic stabilization drills)
Gentle submaximal shoulder isometrics
Continue use of cryotherapy PRN

Weeks 5–6

Restrictions
Discontinue shoulder sling at 6 weeks
Continue no resisted active isolated biceps activity (elbow flexion or forearm supination x 6 weeks)
No biceps loading until week 10
Continue no active ER, extension, or elevation

Protocol
Continue to gradually improve ROM
Flexion and Scaption to 145^0 (can progress further if tolerated)
ER to 50^0
IR to 60^0
Full ROM should be achieved at 8–10weeks
Initiate limited AROM/AAROM of shoulder to 90^0 flexion or abduction
Continue submaximal shoulder isometrics
Can begin AROM supination (no resistance/elbow flexed)

Clinical milestones to progress to Phase II
Flexion to 125^0 (can progress further if tolerated)
Abduction to 70^0
Scapular plane IR to 40^0
ER to 40^0

Fig. 2. (*A–C*) Adapted Postoperative SLAP tear Rehabilitation Protocol. (*From* Manske R, Prohaska D. Superior labrum anterior to posterior (SLAP) rehabilitation in the overhead athlete. *Phys Ther Sport Off J Assoc Chart Physiother Sports Med*. 2010;11(4):110-121. https://doi.org/10.1016/j.ptsp.2010.06.004.)

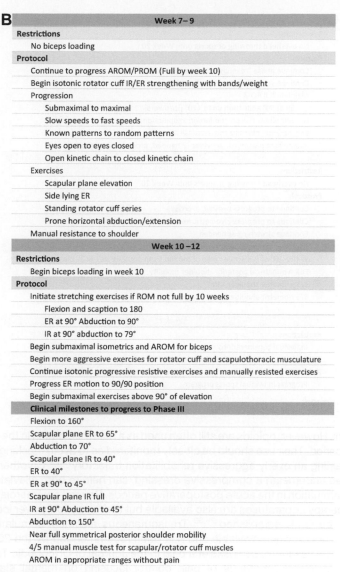

B	Week 7– 9
Restrictions	
No biceps loading	
Protocol	
Continue to progress AROM/PROM (Full by week 10)	
Begin isotonic rotator cuff IR/ER strengthening with bands/weight	
Progression	
Submaximal to maximal	
Slow speeds to fast speeds	
Known patterns to random patterns	
Eyes open to eyes closed	
Open kinetic chain to closed kinetic chain	
Exercises	
Scapular plane elevation	
Side lying ER	
Standing rotator cuff series	
Prone horizontal abduction/extension	
Manual resistance to shoulder	

Week 10 –12	
Restrictions	
Begin biceps loading in week 10	
Protocol	
Initiate stretching exercises if ROM not full by 10 weeks	
Flexion and scaption to 180	
ER at 90° Abduction to 90°	
IR at 90° abduction to 79°	
Begin submaximal isometrics and AROM for biceps	
Begin more aggressive exercises for rotator cuff and scapulothoracic musculature	
Continue isotonic progressive resistive exercises and manually resisted exercises	
Progress ER motion to 90/90 position	
Begin submaximal exercises above 90° of elevation	

Clinical milestones to progress to Phase III
Flexion to 160°
Scapular plane ER to 65°
Abduction to 70°
Scapular plane IR to 40°
ER to 40°
ER at 90° to 45°
Scapular plane IR full
IR at 90° Abduction to 45°
Abduction to 150°
Near full symmetrical posterior shoulder mobility
4/5 manual muscle test for scapular/rotator cuff muscles
AROM in appropriate ranges without pain

Fig. 2. (*Continued*)

also be used for comparison throughout the rehabilitation process. Dominant versus nondominant limb differences may be considered with regards to comparative strength and stability. Additional sports-specific therapy may be required to achieve desired goals, especially for elite athletes.[26]

Pharmacologic or Medical Treatment Options

Pain management is an integral part of the postoperative rehabilitation process. Pain may be a valuable indicator during the rehabilitative process, guiding functional progression.[27,28]

During rehabilitation, scheduled non-steroidal anti-inflammatory drugs (NSAIDs), both topical and oral, along with acetaminophen form the basis of pharmacologic

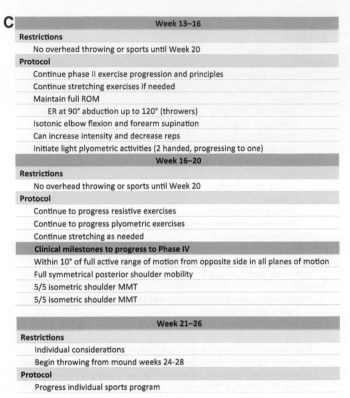

C

Week 13–16
Restrictions
No overhead throwing or sports until Week 20
Protocol
Continue phase II exercise progression and principles
Continue stretching exercises if needed
Maintain full ROM
ER at 90° abduction up to 120° (throwers)
Isotonic elbow flexion and forearm supination
Can increase intensity and decrease reps
Initiate light plyometric activities (2 handed, progressing to one)
Week 16–20
Restrictions
No overhead throwing or sports until Week 20
Protocol
Continue to progress resistive exercises
Continue to progress plyometric exercises
Continue stretching as needed
Clinical milestones to progress to Phase IV
Within 10° of full active range of motion from opposite side in all planes of motion
Full symmetrical posterior shoulder mobility
5/5 isometric shoulder MMT
5/5 isometric shoulder MMT
Week 21–26
Restrictions
Individual considerations
Begin throwing from mound weeks 24-28
Protocol
Progress individual sports program

Fig. 2. (*Continued*)

pain control. However, opioids are still often used as a pain medication in the early postoperative period. Their use should be closely monitored as to avoid masking excessive pain suggesting an overly aggressive rehabilitation trajectory[28,29] Cryotherapy, using ice wrapped underneath a compressive dressing, can help to both alleviate pain and reduce inflammation in the acute postoperative periods. Several commercial compressive cryotherapy apparatuses are also available but their superiority over ice wrapping has yet to be firmly established.[28,30] Transcutaneous electrical stimulation is also an effective option when available and has been recommended by the 2019 clinical practice guidelines for musculoskeletal pain in the Journal of Orthopedic Trauma.[28]

Other nontraditional methods of pain control focusing on mental state can be included into the rehabilitative process. Although the evidence to support many of these interventions is still in the investigational stage, the low cost and potential benefit make them an attractive adjunct therapy. Meditation, mental imagery, music, and aromatherapy are recommended to patients throughout rehabilitation.[31] Gentle massage may also be incorporated; however, it should be performed or specified by the supervising physical therapist to avoid manipulation or damage to the surgical repair.

Rehabilitation Protocol

A suggested protocol is templated as a 26-week return to function guide, divided into 4 phases (**Fig. 2**A–D). It is based on the method originally described by Maske and Prohaska in *Physical Therapy in Sport*.[6] A variation of this protocol is used by surgeons throughout the country.[25] It begins with a protective phase focusing on allowing the repair to heal with minimal stress. Stress is gradually introduced in the moderation protection phase, and the subsequent minimum protection phase. Finally, the advanced strengthening phase ends the protocol. Although the protocol is templated at 26 weeks, there are specific milestones that patients must meet before procession to the next phase. If a patient has not met their milestones at the templated week, it is recommended to continue in the current phase until they do. Graded progression may be dictated by surgical repair.

Protective Phase (Day 1 to Week 6)

The goals of this phase are to

- Maintain integrity of the repair
- Control pain
- Reduce inflammation
- Counter the effect of immobilization
- Decrease atrophy
- Promote stability of the shoulder

Formal rehabilitation generally begins during the first week postoperatively (see **Fig. 2**A). Patients with a protracted preoperative course and others with concerns for contracture or stiffness may be instructed to begin earlier. The intent of this phase is to minimize any tension on the repair while preventing adhesion of the capsule and ensuring diffusion of nutrients is possible throughout the joint. Recommended immobilization time ranges from 4 to 6 weeks.[25] The risk of adhesion, stiffness, and atrophy with 6 weeks of sling usage is weighed against premature stress and possible failure of the repair. In addition to reducing gravity-mediated stress on the repair, a sling may help to prevent premature tensioning and active engagement of the biceps tendon. Simultaneously during rehabilitation, a gradual increase in passive range of motion (PROM), active-assisted range of motion, and active range of motion (AROM) help prevent stiffness. Various isometric exercises and rhythmic stabilization also help to promote shoulder stability and proprioception while minimizing activation of the biceps (**Fig. 3**).[32] Specific emphasis is placed on mobilization of the posterior capsule as tightness in this region has been proposed as a risk factor of SLAP tears.[6,33]

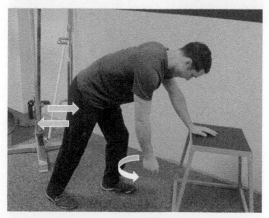

Fig. 3. Codman's exercise is a great way to achieve early range of motion without stress on the repair. During this maneuver, the patient hangs the injured arms and passively rotates the limb by moving the hips and torso.

Moderate Protection Phase (Weeks 7–12)

The goals of this phase are to

- Restore range of motion by week 10
- Continue to maintain the integrity of the repair
- Begin strength and balance training of rotator cuff

This phase builds on the range of motion developed in phase I and works toward full range of motion by week 10, with a continued emphasis on maintain the integrity of the repair (see **Fig. 2**B). Patients who have plateau or have difficulty making the clinical milestone from the previous phase may require aggressive mobilization techniques; however, this should be the minority of patients. Joint mobilization (**Fig. 4**) in addition to stretching (**Fig. 5**) has been shown to be effective for patients with residual posterior capsule tightness.[34] Now, strength training begins with emphasis on balance in the rotator cuff (**Fig. 6**) and week 10 introduces gradual activation of the biceps. Lower body and core training should continue to ensure patients maintain previous levels of strength, endurance, and coordination.

Minimum Protection Phase (Weeks 13–20)

The goals of this phase are to

- Full AROM/PROM without pain
- Restoration of muscle strength, power, and endurance
- No pain or tenderness
- Gradual initiation of functional activities

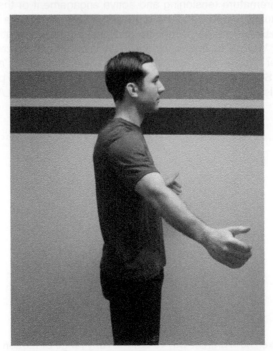

Fig. 4. Mobilization in the scapular plane optimally aligns the glenoid and humeral head, reducing impingement.

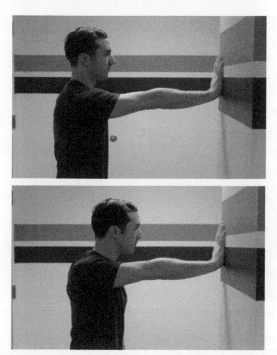

Fig. 5. The scapular wall press allows for mobilization of the scapula without stress on the repair.

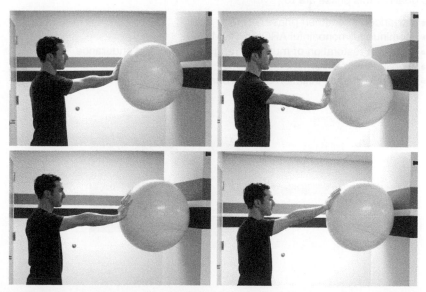

Fig. 6. Rhythmic stabilization drills can be performed with a partner or independent with an aid as above. This method supports the limb, minimizing stress on the repair, while focusing on proprioceptive training.

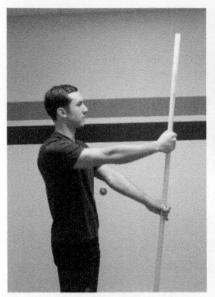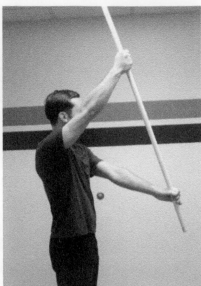

Fig. 7. Passive range of motion is essential to prevent adhesion and stiffness.

This focus of this phase is continued strength training and motion without pain (see **Fig. 2**C). Any adhesive or fibrosed tissue should be eliminated through stretching and mobilization (**Figs. 7** and **8**). Overhead throwing is held until week 20 due to the unique stress this motion places of the labrum.

Advanced Strengthen Phase (Weeks 21–26)

The goals of this phase are to

- Advanced strengthen phase
- Continue full nonpainful AROM/PROM
- Continue restoration of muscle strength, power, and endurance
- Continue no pain or tenderness
- Continue gradual initiation of functional activities

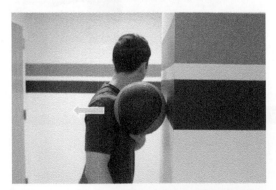

Fig. 8. Posterior translation of the humeral head through manual manipulation or self-guided therapy as above can increase posterior capsule mobility. Such mobility is thought to be a protective factor against further damage to the labrum.

Patients in the phase continue to maintain range of motion and build their strength and conditioning back to preinjury levels (see **Fig. 2**D). The exact exercises should be individualized to the patient. Overhead throwers should gradually increase the throwing distance and projectile weight. Nonthrowers who experienced a traction or compression injury may not require as much of an emphasis on mechanics, and instead work to increase other motions such as pressing, pulling, or rowing.

Ending the Protocol and Return to Play Considerations

Perhaps the most challenging aspect of SLAP tear rehabilitation is the question of when a patient can return to full competitive play. Although certain populations such as those aged older than 40 years and overhead athletes are more challenging to return to their preinjury level of competitiveness, there is no predictable set of risk factors that identify the individual patient who may have a less than optimal outcome.[5,6,19] Several objective criteria have been described to guide the clinical decision of when to no longer limit the activities of a postoperative patient.[10,24,35,36] Perhaps, the most comprehensive is the "3 P Program: Performance, Practice, and Play" described by Wilk and colleagues.[10] Quality of life metrics such as the Western Ontario Shoulder Instability Index [37] or the Kerlan-Jobe Orthopedic Clinic[38] score can also help guide the decision. However, the universal application of any metric has not been well studied. In any case, the decision should not be guided purely by time since the operative repair and instead should focus on the functional status and occupational demands of the patient.

In absence of a checklist that "clears" patients for return to play, there are criteria that patients should meet before returning to high-level function.

1. Return of full or near full range (>90%) of motion (**Fig. 9**)
2. Return of at least 80% of the preinjury level of strength or speed

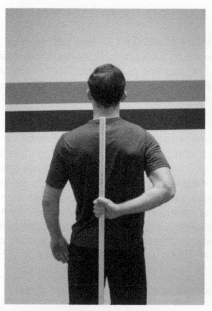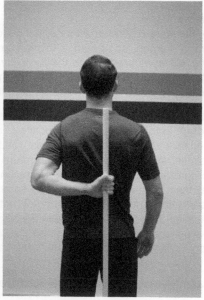

Fig. 9. Comparison of range of motion to the uninjured side is a critical component of return to play criteria.

3. Pain-free submaximal play
4. Completion of an activity/sport specific ramp-up program

Some patients may return to play too early and experience pain or discomfort in excess of expected soreness. Such incidence should result in prompt evaluation by the surgical and physical therapy teams.

Special Populations

Overhead athletes

Overhead athletes are a challenging population to treat, with the lowest return to play rate.[9,11,23,24] The biomechanics of overhead throwing involves hyperabduction and external rotation, which place high levels of stress on the labrum and biceps tendon. After repair, these forces will continue to affect the surgical site, making reinjury or chronic pain a possibility. Due to this fact, these patients require the most gradual return to play as well as an emphasis on posterior capsule mobility, scapular stabilization exercises, and improved endurance. Michener and colleagues[24] outline progressing to a throwing program at approximately 16 weeks postoperatively, with goals of return to sport at 24 weeks. Limited internal rotation and a tight posterior capsule have been hypothesized to increase compressive forces on the superior labrum.[7,39] Similarly, muscle fatigue may limit proprioception and thereby alters throwing mechanics.[40] To combat this, Wilk and colleagues[41] endorse a "throwers ten" exercise program, which provides a framework for endurance training of the shoulder, scapulothoracic joint, trunk, and lower extremity. This program, or a similar emphasis on endurance, should be incorporated into the advanced strengthening phase of the rehabilitation process. A critical analysis of throwing mechanics as the athlete is returning to full activity offers the opportunity to improve form and reduce risk of reinjury. The goal of functional rehabilitation is to gradually reintroduce sport-specific motions, positions, and forces. Specifically, postrehabilitation functional testing may be used to evaluate readiness to return to sport.

Female athletes

Prior literature has reported a greater incidence of shoulder injuries and overuse injuries in women, compared with men, overhead athletes.[42–45] Women commonly score higher with regards to the flexibility components on the functional movement system compared with men.[42] Due to these functional differences, modified sex-specific guidelines may prove to be pertinent.

Postoperative complications. SLAP repairs are a technically demanding surgery, and although outcomes overall are positive, complications may occur.[22] Patients may experience residual pain or stiffness, rotator cuff defects, articular cartilage injuries, persistent synovitis, or suboptimal return to competitive play.[3] If rehabilitation fails to progress functional recovery, it is recommended that the patient return to the surgical team for evaluation. Although soreness and discomfort are expected during rehabilitation, sudden loss of range of motion or extensive pain also requires prompt evaluation. True SLAP repair failure is likely multifactorial and requires the evaluation of an experienced surgeon.[2,22] Some patients ultimately may require revision but a recent review of national insurance database found this to be uncommon (<3%).[46]

SUMMARY/DISCUSSION/FUTURE DIRECTIONS

Since SLAP repairs were first described more than 3 decades ago, they remain a challenging entity to diagnose, treat, and subsequently manage. No high-quality clinical trials exist to identify the best postoperative rehabilitation protocol. Nevertheless, the protocol described in this article is based on a thorough understanding of pathoanatomy, physiology, and clinical experience. It has demonstrated success in clinical practice, and it provides an excellent framework to return patients to their preinjury competitive level and allows for individual variation and attention. The ultimate decision of when to return to competitive play is a challenging one that must consider objective and subjective criteria, as well as occupation demands.

CLINICS CARE POINTS

- Postoperative rehabilitation following a SLAP repair is guided by the principle of gradual return to preinjury function while preserving the integrity of the surgical repair.
- Objective criteria can be used to gradually progress individuals through a postoperative rehabilitation protocol.
- A majority of individuals will successfully return to sport-specific or occupation-specific activities.

DISCLOSURE

The authors have nothing to disclose.

REFERENCES

1. Andrews JR, Carson WG, McLeod WD. Glenoid labrum tears related to the long head of the biceps. Am J Sports Med 1985;13(5):337–41.
2. Snyder SJ, Karzel RP, Pizzo WD, et al. SLAP lesions of the shoulder. Arthroscopy 1990;6(4):274–9.
3. Weber SC, Martin DF, Seiler JG, et al. Superior labrum anterior and posterior lesions of the shoulder: incidence rates, complications, and outcomes as reported by american board of orthopedic surgery part II candidates. Am J Sports Med 2012;40(7):1538–43.
4. Onyekwelu I, Khatib O, Zuckerman JD, et al. The rising incidence of arthroscopic superior labrum anterior and posterior (SLAP) repairs. J Shoulder Elbow Surg 2012;21(6):728–31.
5. Zhang AL, Kreulen C, Ngo SS, et al. Demographic trends in arthroscopic SLAP repair in the United States. Am J Sports Med 2012;40(5):1144–7.
6. Manske R, Prohaska D. Superior labrum anterior to posterior (SLAP) rehabilitation in the overhead athlete. Phys Ther Sport Off J Assoc Chart Physiother Sports Med 2010;11(4):110–21.
7. Kibler WB, Kuhn JE, Wilk K, et al. The disabled throwing shoulder: spectrum of pathology—10-year update. Arthrosc J Arthrosc Relat Surg 2013;29(1): 141–61.e26.
8. Kibler WB, Sciascia A. Current practice for the surgical treatment of SLAP lesions: a systematic review. Arthrosc J Arthrosc Relat Surg 2016;32(4):669–83.
9. Brockmeier SF, Voos JE, Williams RJ, et al. Outcomes after arthroscopic repair of type-II SLAP lesions. J Bone Joint Surg Am 2009;91(7):1595–603.
10. Wilk KE, Bagwell MS, Davies GJ, et al. Return to sport participation criteria following shoulder injury: a clinical commentary. Int J Sports Phys Ther 2020; 15(4):624–42.

11. Gorantla K, Gill C, Wright RW. The outcome of type II SLAP repair: a systematic review. Arthroscopy 2010;26(4):537–45.

12. Erickson J, Lavery K, Monica J, et al. Surgical treatment of symptomatic superior labrum anterior-posterior tears in patients older than 40 years: a systematic review. Am J Sports Med 2015;43(5):1274–82.

13. Patterson BM, Creighton RA, Spang JT, et al. Surgical trends in the treatment of superior labrum anterior and posterior lesions of the shoulder: analysis of data from the american board of orthopaedic surgery certification examination database. Am J Sports Med 2014;42(8):1904–10.

14. Maffet MW, Gartsman GM, Moseley B. Superior labrum-biceps tendon complex lesions of the shoulder. Am J Sports Med 1995;23(1):93–8.

15. Gartsman GM, Hammerman SM. Superior labrum, anterior and posterior lesions: when and how to treat them. Clin Sports Med 2000;19(1):115–24.

16. Morgan CD, Burkhart SS, Palmeri M, et al. Type II SLAP lesions: three subtypes and their relationships to superior instability and rotator cuff tears. Arthrosc J Arthrosc Relat Surg 1998;14(6):553–65.

17. Powell SE, Nord KD, Ryu RKN. The diagnosis, classification, and treatment of SLAP lesions. Oper Tech Sports Med 2012;20(1):46–56.

18. Harris JD. Editorial Commentary: On Kibler & Sciascia: What Did the Five Fingers Say to the Face? SLAP. A Systematic Review Wake-Up Call to Improve SLAP Repair Guidelines. Arthrosc J Arthrosc Relat Surg 2016;32(4):684–5.

19. Kim TK, Queale WS, Cosgarea AJ, et al. Clinical features of the different types of SLAP lesions: an analysis of one hundred and thirty-nine cases. J Bone Joint Surg Am 2003;85(1):66–71.

20. Hegedus EJ, Goode AP, Cook CE, et al. Which physical examination tests provide clinicians with the most value when examining the shoulder? Update of a systematic review with meta-analysis of individual tests. Br J Sports Med 2012; 46(14):964–78.

21. Meserve BB, Cleland JA, Boucher TR. A meta-analysis examining clinical test utility for assessing superior labral anterior posterior lesions. Am J Sports Med 2009; 37(11):2252–8.

22. Werner BC, Brockmeier SF, Miller MD. Etiology, diagnosis, and management of failed SLAP repair. J Am Acad Orthop Surg 2014;22(9):554–65.

23. Neuman BJ, Boisvert CB, Reiter B, et al. Results of arthroscopic repair of type II superior labral anterior posterior lesions in overhead athletes: assessment of return to preinjury playing level and satisfaction. Am J Sports Med 2011;39(9): 1883–8.

24. Michener LA, Abrams JS, Bliven KCH, et al. National athletic trainers' association position statement: evaluation, management, and outcomes of and return-to- play criteria for overhead athletes with superior labral anterior-posterior injuries. J Athl Train 2018;53(3):209–29.

25. Hermanns CA, Coda RG, Cheema S, et al. Variability in rehabilitation protocols after superior labrum anterior posterior surgical repair. Kans J Med 2021;14: 243–8.

26. Yung PSH, Fong DTP, Kong MF, et al. Arthroscopic repair of isolated type II superior labrum anterior-posterior lesion. Knee Surg Sports Traumatol Arthrosc 2008;16(12):1151–7.

27. Taylor J, Taylor S. Pain education and management in the rehabilitation from sports injury. Sport Psychol 1998;12(1):68–88.

28. Hsu JR, Mir H, Wally MK, et al. Orthopaedic trauma association musculoskeletal pain task force. clinical practice guidelines for pain management in acute musculoskeletal injury. J Orthop Trauma 2019;33(5):e158–82.

29. Koehler RM, Okoroafor UC, Cannada LK. A systematic review of opioid use after extremity trauma in orthopedic surgery. Injury 2018;49(6):1003–7.

30. Kraeutler MJ, Reynolds KA, Long C, et al. Compressive cryotherapy versus ice-a prospective, randomized study on postoperative pain in patients undergoing arthroscopic rotator cuff repair or subacromial decompression. J Shoulder Elbow Surg 2015;24(6):854–9.

31. Fan M, Chen Z. A systematic review of non-pharmacological interventions used for pain relief after orthopedic surgical procedures. Exp Ther Med 2020;20(5):1.

32. Cools AM, Borms D, Cottens S, et al. Rehabilitation exercises for athletes with biceps disorders and SLAP lesions: a continuum of exercises with increasing loads on the biceps. Am J Sports Med 2014;42(6):1315–22.

33. Wilk KE, Macrina LC. Nonoperative and postoperative rehabilitation for injuries of the throwing shoulder. Sports Med Arthrosc Rev 2014;22(2):137–50.

34. Manske RC, Meschke M, Porter A, et al. A randomized controlled single-blinded comparison of stretching versus stretching and joint mobilization for posterior shoulder tightness measured by internal rotation motion loss. Sports Health 2010;2(2):94–100.

35. Enad JG, Gaines RJ, White SM, et al. Arthroscopic superior labrum anterior-posterior repair in military patients. J Shoulder Elbow Surg 2007;16(3):300–5.

36. Sayde WM, Cohen SB, Ciccotti MG, et al. Return to play after type II superior labral anterior-posterior lesion repairs in athletes: a systematic review. Clin Orthop Relat Res 2012;470(6):1595–600.

37. Kirkley A, Griffin S, McLintock H, Ng L. The development and evaluation of a disease-specific quality of life measurement tool for shoulder instability the western ontario shoulder instability index (WOSI. Am J Sports Med 1998;26:764–72.

38. Alberta FG, ElAttrache NS, Bissell S, et al. The development and validation of a functional assessment tool for the upper extremity in the overhead athlete. Am J Sports Med 2010;38(5):903–11.

39. Knesek M, Skendzel JG, Dines JS, et al. Diagnosis and management of superior labral anterior posterior tears in throwing athletes. Am J Sports Med 2013;41(2):444–60.

40. Carpenter JE, Blasier RB, Pellizzon GG. The effects of muscle fatigue on shoulder joint position sense. Am J Sports Med 1998;26(2):262–5.

41. Wilk KE, Yenchak AJ, Arrigo CA, et al. The Advanced Throwers Ten Exercise Program: a new exercise series for enhanced dynamic shoulder control in the overhead throwing athlete. Phys Sportsmed 2011;39(4):90–7.

42. Chimera NJ, Smith CA, Warren M. Injury history, sex, and performance on the functional movement screen and Y balance test. J Athl Train 2015;50:475–85.

43. O'Connor S, Huseyin OR, Whyte EF, et al. A 2-year prospective study of injuries and illness in an elite national junior tennis program. Phys Sportsmed 2020;48:342–8.

44. Vincent HK, Zdziarski LA, Vincent KR. Review of lacrosse-related musculoskeletal injuries in high school and collegiate players. Sports Health 2015;7:448–51.

45. Boudrea S, Mattes L, Lowenstein N, et al. Customizing functional rehabilitation and return to sport in the female overhead athlete. Rehabil Return Sport Athletes 2022;4(1):E271–85.
46. Taylor SA, Degen RM, White AE, et al. Risk factors for revision surgery after superior labral anterior-posterior repair: a national perspective. Am J Sports Med 2017;45(7):1640–4.

Physical Therapy for the Treatment of Shoulder Instability

Daniel J. Stokes, MD, Timothy P. McCarthy, MD,
Rachel M. Frank, MD*

KEYWORDS

- Rehabilitation • Glenohumeral joint • Instability • Physical therapy

KEY POINTS

- The glenohumeral joint is the joint most prone to instability in the body.
- Shoulder instability is the separation of the humeral head from the glenoid fossa.
- The goal of rehabilitation is to restore pain-free mobility, strength, and functioning.
- Rehabilitation improves functional status, strength, and scapular positioning.

INTRODUCTION

Glenohumeral joint (GHJ) instability is the separation of the humeral head from the glenoid fossa. The unique anatomy of the shoulder allows for the most range of motion (ROM) of any joint in the body.[1] However, this wide ROM increases the susceptibility to instability.

The GHJ is the most dislocated joint in the body, representing 50% of all major joint dislocations,[2] with an incidence rate of 23.9 cases per 100,000.[3] The incidence of shoulder instability in college and high school athletes makes up 0.12 and .22 instability events per 1000 athlete exposures, respectively.[4] The highest risk demographic for GHJ instability are young athletes in their second and third decades of life.[5] It is essential to understand the mechanism and the appropriate management to ensure a return of full shoulder function, prevention of recurrence, and a quick return to play (RTP).

ANATOMY

Shoulder instability severity ranges from subluxation to dislocation.[5] Knowing the anatomy of the GHJ is imperative for understanding the causes of shoulder instability. Laxity is classified as anterior, posterior, or multidirectional shoulder instability.

Department of Orthopedic Surgery, University of Colorado School of Medicine, Aurora, CO, USA
* Corresponding author. Department of Orthopaedic Surgery, UCHealth CU Sports Medicine - Colorado Center, 2000 South Colorado Boulevard, Tower 1, Suite 4500, Denver, CO 80222.
E-mail address: rachel.frank@cuanschutz.edu

Phys Med Rehabil Clin N Am 34 (2023) 393–408
https://doi.org/10.1016/j.pmr.2022.12.006
1047-9651/23/© 2022 Elsevier Inc. All rights reserved.
pmr.theclinics.com

Table 1	
Functions of static stabilizers	
Structure	**Function**
Rotator interval	Restrains posteroinferior translation in adduction
Joint capsule	Encloses the GHJ and creates a seal providing negative intra-articular pressure (suction effect)
Coracohumeral ligament	Extra-articular; restraint against posterior translation (FF, IR) and inferior translation (adduction, ER)
Superior glenohumeral ligament	Primary restraint against inferior translation in adduction; acts as a pulley for the LHBT
Middle glenohumeral ligament	Resists anterior translation in ER with 45° of abduction
Inferior glenohumeral ligament	Primary restraint against anteroinferior translation
Anterior band	Primary restraint against anterior translation in 90° abduction and ER
Posterior band	Primary restraint against posterior translation in 90° abduction

Abbreviations: ER, external rotation; FF, forward flexion; IR, internal rotation; LHBT, long head of the bicep tendon.

The unique bony articulation between the humeral head and the glenoid fossa provides a wide degree of motion and inherent instability. The glenoid fossa is pear-shaped, retroverted, and shallow.[6] The size of the humeral head compared with the glenoid is incongruent, commonly equated to a golf ball sitting on a golf tee. This 4:1 ratio in surface area between the humeral head and glenoid provides minimal bony constraint and unrestricted movement throughout the joint.[7] Though there is a discrepancy in bone surfaces between the glenoid and humerus, the articulating cartilage surface area is congruent, creating an inherently stable GHJ where small translations of the humeral head on the glenoid are considered normal.[8] Damage to the articulating surfaces results in more extensive pathologic translations.

The GHJ receives stabilization from both static and dynamic stabilizers. **Table 1** describes the role of the rotator interval, the glenohumeral ligaments, and the glenoid labrum.[1] Each structure is critical in providing passive stabilization to the GHJ.

The coordination of dynamic muscle forces further stabilizes the shoulder. The deltoid, biceps brachii, rotator cuff, and periscapular muscles provide dynamic stabilization by maintaining contact between the humeral head and the center of the glenoid surface.[9] Each component contributes to maintaining proper shoulder stability and overall function.

PATHOPHYSIOLOGICAL MECHANISMS
Anterior Shoulder Instability

Anterior shoulder instability (ASI) is the pathologic laxity of the GHJ in the anterior direction. It is the most common shoulder instability, accounting for over 90% of cases.[10] The most common mechanism of injury resulting in ASI is a force on an abducted, flexed, and externally rotated arm.

When the humeral head is displaced anteriorly, the natural tendency is to retract, resulting in impaction of the posterior humeral head on the anteroinferior glenoid. A

Bankart lesion is an avulsion of the anteroinferior labrum from the glenoid rim. A bony Bankart lesion, or anteroinferior glenoid rim fracture, can occur.[11] A Hill-Sachs lesion is a chondral impaction of the posterosuperior humeral head secondary to contact with the anterior glenoid rim. Bankart lesions often result in recurrent instability.

Posterior Shoulder Instability

Posterior shoulder instability (PSI) is dysfunctional laxity posteriorly and is the second most prevalent, accounting for approximately 2% to 5% of cases.[12] PSI typically has a subtle onset, with pain being the primary complaint.[13] Partially attributed to this discrepancy are the differences in ligamentous support provided by the IGHL.

The anterior band of the IGHL is a strong band of tissue that is the primary restraint against the humerus displacing forward.[14] The posterior band of the IGHL limits posterior displacement but is significantly thinner in comparison. In a healthy shoulder, this band is sufficient. However, repetitive micro-trauma to the posterior band, primarily in a forward flexed, adducted, and internally rotated arm, causes PSI.[15]

Articulating surfaces play a vital role in posterior stability. Therefore, glenoid hypoplasia and excessive retroversion predispose an individual to recurrent PSI.[16] Retroversion of the glenoid increases humerus external rotation (ER).[15] The average retroversion of the glenoid is $1° \pm 3°$.[17] There is a strong correlation between the amount of glenoid retroversion and the risk of recurrent PSI.[18,19]

Table 2 highlights labral and humeral head characteristic lesions found in PSI.

Multidirectional Shoulder Instability

Multidirectional instability (MDI) of the shoulder is symptomatic laxity of the GHJ in more than one direction.[20] MDI can occur in the setting of connective tissue disorders, a single traumatic event, or repetitive microtrauma.

Hyperlaxity alone does not meet the requirements for MDI but can increase the risk. Instability requires the presence of symptoms commonly reported as nonspecific pain, weakness, or declining athletic performance, in addition to an abnormal translation of the shoulder.[21] Owing to the hypermobile nature of connective tissue disorders, individuals with Marfan and Ehlers-Danlos syndromes are at increased risk of developing MDI.[22]

The most common etiology is microtrauma caused by repetitive movements. Overhead athletes such as volleyball players, gymnasts, climbers, and weightlifters sustain repetitive microtrauma resulting in structural damage to the static and dynamic stabilizers. These patients present with an insidious onset. However, a sizable labral tear may be present when the injury is a single traumatic event.

Characteristic findings shown on imaging can support an MDI diagnosis. The presence of a patulous or redundant inferior capsule on MRI may be indicative of MDI.

Table 2	
Posterior shoulder instability characteristic lesions	
Lesion	**Description**
Reverse Hill-Sachs	Erosion of the anteromedial aspect of the humeral head
Reverse Bankart	Posteroinferior labral detachment
Reverse Bony Bankart	Bony avulsion of the posterior glenoid rim
Kim	Posterior labral tear between an intact superficial labrum and glenoid articular cartilage

EVALUATION/INDICATIONS FOR TREATMENT
Physical Examination

A detailed history can help guide the physical examination. The interview should address the mechanism of injury, location of pain, first-time dislocation, frequency of instability events, avoidance of provocative positions, and any repetitive movements or overhead activities. Regardless of suspected ASI, PSI, or MDI, every shoulder examination should include bilateral inspection, palpation, active/passive ROM, strength, and neurovascular testing. It is also important to evaluate the cervical spine during shoulder examination.

SPECIAL TESTING FOR INSTABILITY
Anterior Shoulder Instability Special Tests

- Anterior drawer: With the patient sitting upright and the arm relaxed by the side, the examiner will place an index finger on the coracoid process with the thumb at the scapular spine. While grasping the humeral head, an anterior force is applied. This test is positive if greater than 50% of the humeral head translates anteriorly beyond the glenoid rim.[17]
- Anterior load and shift: With the patient supine and the shoulder at 40° to 60° of abduction and forward flexion, the examiner will put an axial load on the humerus, centering it within the glenoid. An anterior force to the humeral head is applied, causing an anterior shift. Increased translation compared with the contralateral side suggests ASI.[23]
- Apprehension/Relocation/Release test:
  - With the patient supine on the edge of the examination bed and the shoulder at 90° of abduction, the examiner will gently externally rotate the arm to 90°. If the patient reports pain or apprehension, the test is positive.
  - With the shoulder at 90° of abduction and ER, the examiner will apply a posterior force to the humerus. If positive, the patient will report decreased apprehension.
  - The examiner withdraws the posterior force on the proximal humerus from the relocation position. This test is positive if the patient reports a return of pain or apprehension[24] (**Figs. 1** and **2**).

Posterior Shoulder Instability Special Tests

- Posterior drawer: This is the same maneuver as the anterior drawer, but a posterior force is applied.[17]
- Posterior load and shift: This is the same maneuver as anterior load and shift, but a posterior force to the humeral head is applied, causing it to shift posteriorly.[23]
- Jerk test: With the patient sitting upright and the arm at 90° of forward flexion and internal rotation with full adduction, the examiner will apply a posterior force at the elbow while looking for subluxation. The examiner will then abduct the arm while maintaining the posterior load. As the humeral head relocates, a clunk indicates a posterior labral tear.[16]
- Kim test: With the patient sitting upright and the shoulder at 90° of abduction and ~45° of forward flexion, the examiner will apply an axial load on the elbow while simultaneously applying a posterior force on the humerus, looking for subluxation. Pain or a clunk indicates a positive test[16] (**Fig. 3**).

Multidirectional Instability Special Tests

- Sulcus sign: With the patient in a standing position and the arm relaxed by the side, the examiner will apply a downward force on the arm while observing the

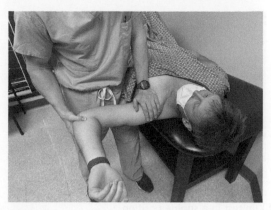

Fig. 1. Apprehension test.

superior aspect of the humeral head for an interval of >1 to 2 cm. When the sulcus sign remains positive in ER, this indicates rotator interval incompetence.[20]

- Gagey/hyperabduction test: With the patient sitting upright and the arm relaxed by the side, the examiner will stabilize the shoulder by placing an index finger on the clavicle with the thumb at the scapular spine. The examiner will then passively abduct the arm while preventing shoulder elevation. This test is positive if the end range is > 105° abduction and indicates laxity of the IGHL **(Fig. 4)**.
- Beighton score: Components of screening for hyperlaxity include:
  - Passive apposition of the thumb to the forearm (2 points)
  - Passive hyperextension of the fifth metacarpophalangeal joint greater than 90° (2 points)
  - Passive hyperextension of the elbow greater than 10° (2 points)
  - Active hyperextension of the knee greater than 10° (2 points)
  - Active forward flexion at the waist, placing the palms of the hand on the floor with the knees fully extended (1 point)

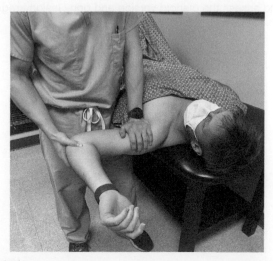

Fig. 2. Relocation test.

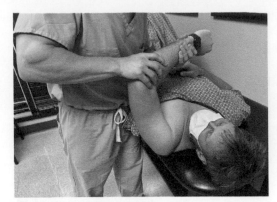

Fig. 3. Variation of Kim test in a supine position.

Values > 4 indicate a positive Beighton score suggesting joint hyperlaxity.[25]

Instability can show positive findings from each subset. For this reason, it is essential to manage each patient on a case-by-case basis. If surgery is elected, each physical examination finding should be confirmed and compared with the contralateral side under anesthesia before the operation.[17]

IMAGING

The first imaging modality for a patient with suspected GHJ instability should be plain film radiographs. The standard series should include an anteroposterior (AP), a true AP (Grashey view), axillary, and modified scapular Y views. Specialty views, such as the Stryker notch and West Point view, provide insight into Hill-Sachs defect and anteroinferior glenoid rim fracture.

MRI assesses soft-tissue damage in all patients. Magnetic resonance arthrography (MRA), or an MRI with contrast enhancement, can increase the sensitivity to the capsuloligamentous complex. This study can be helpful in PSI to evaluate a Kim lesion or in MDI to check for a patulous capsule.[16] Computed tomography should measure glenoid bone loss and assess the glenoid version and bony lesion irregularities.[26]

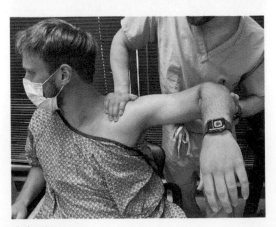

Fig. 4. Gagey/hyperabduction test.

Although shoulder instability is a clinical diagnosis, imaging can contribute to and enhance subsequent management options.[26] Managing shoulder instability should encompass subjective considerations and patient preference. A physical rehabilitation program has proven to improve outcomes, regardless of conservative or surgical management.

TREATMENT

Treatment of shoulder instability is multi-faceted. Patient-specific goals and risk stratification of adverse outcomes require a collaborative effort between medical specialists and the patient to provide comprehensive options and informed decision-making.[27] Options for treatment can include an initial course of physical therapy versus early surgical intervention. Surgical intervention followed by physical therapy should be considered with risk factors associated with a high recurrence rate or previously failed conservative management. Risk factors that might prompt the decision for surgical intervention include:

Age: A patient's age upon the initial subluxation/dislocation is predictive of recurrent instability. Compared with arthroscopic stabilization, conservative management in a population less than 26 years of age leads to failure rates as high as 60% to 75%.[28–30] In a study comparing recurrence rate, RTP, and patient-perceived improvement, acute surgical stabilization of first-time shoulder dislocation was found to be more effective than conservative treatment in patients 15 to 25 years of age.[31]

Trauma: Most first-time shoulder dislocations have a traumatic etiology. Repetitive trauma, especially in overhead athletes or high-impact sports, increases the risk for recurrent instability events. Arthroscopic management has resulted in a lower recurrence rate than conservative management and a significantly higher rate of RTP.[32] Therefore, surgery is effective and may be desirable, especially in young male athletes, to reduce the recurrence rate and increase RTP.[28,31–33]

Structural deficit: Bankart lesions are the most common injury following primary shoulder dislocation. Evidence reveals satisfactory subjective function and surgical success rates for isolated Bankart repair.[34] A fracture following primary dislocation or bone erosion changes the normal shoulder biomechanics and decreases articulating surface area. With recurrent instability, glenoid and humeral defects either enlarge or develop at a significantly higher rate.[35] Identifying bipolar bone defects is critical as they strongly predict postoperative failure when unaddressed.[6]

PHYSICAL REHABILITATION

Rehabilitation plays a fundamental role in successful outcomes following shoulder instability. Most first-time shoulder dislocations are treated nonoperatively.[36] The primary goal of rehabilitation is to restore pain-free mobility, strength, control, and activity-specific functioning.[37]

REHABILITATION APPROACH

A patient with an acute shoulder instability event typically presents with pain and guarding. Commonly, the shoulder is internally rotated, subduing the provocative position. Self-limiting activity is implemented to prevent further pain and injury. The initial goal for rehabilitation should focus on reducing pain and inflammation through a period of immobilization.

Immobilization is consistently agreed upon, but the position and duration have been debated. The immobilization period should be limited, typically one to 3 weeks.

Immobilization allows for patient comfort rather than a decreased risk for recurrence, as the evidence fails to show a significant difference.[38] Likewise, immobilization in ER compared with internal rotation is theorized to provide better soft-tissue positioning relative to the glenoid, thereby decreasing the risk of recurrent instability. However, repeated inconsistencies across these studies have failed to show any substantial benefit of ER.[38]

Early passive motion is encouraged and may contribute to healing while decreasing pain. Early movements are restricted to the scapular plane and less than 90° of abduction with rotational movements.[36] Dynamic GHJ stability begins with gentle isometrics and rhythmic closed kinetic chain exercises.[39] Closed kinetic chain exercises ensure shoulder support through hand fixation on a stable surface, facilitating deltoid, rotator cuff, and scapular muscle coactivation, as well as proprioceptive control.[37]

After 4 to 6 weeks, full ROM and strengthening exercises are implemented. Return of full active ROM is expected in this phase through a gradual progression of flexion, ER, and IR exercises with escalating degrees of abduction.[36] Strengthening exercises are introduced, mainly focusing on the rotator cuff and scapular stabilizers. Rotator cuff activation is maximized primarily through resisted flexion, abduction, and ER. Activation of the supraspinatus and infraspinatus through ER helps anteriorly balance the GHJ against pectoralis major forces. Internal rotation can strengthen the subscapularis, but there is equal activation in the pectoralis major.[27] Therefore, it is essential to find the balance of subscapularis strengthening while promoting GHJ stability.

Periscapular strengthening further increases stability. Scapular dyskinesis needs to be addressed early in rehabilitation as it contributes to shoulder pain, decreased muscle strength, and limited ROM.[39] These patients often have a discrepancy in muscle strength across the scapula resulting in an imbalance. Scapular strengthening exercises restore balance through the activation of the weaker muscles. Once balance returns, advanced scapular strength exercises integrate activity-dependent movements and control.[40]

Resistance, movement complexity, and endurance continue to intensify as the patient progresses. A deliberate rehabilitation program with attention to scapular positioning, dynamic strengthening, and GHJ motion requires a dedicated patient and attentive medical team but ultimately provides optimal outcomes and sustainability with nonoperative management. Jaggi and Alexander[37] outline an exercise-specific rehabilitation protocol for shoulder instability.

POSTERIOR SHOULDER INSTABILITY REHABILITATION

The most common etiology for PSI is subtle onset with pain. Conservative management is typically the primary option in an atraumatic presentation, as bony deformity is often absent.

The insidious onset of pain without an acute trauma does not warrant an immobilization period. Posterior shoulder rehabilitation emphasizes rotator cuff and scapular musculature strengthening, similar to ASI, as these are the primary dynamic stabilizers. A common finding in PSI is downward scapular rotation improved through elevation maneuvers. Though subscapularis strengthening has limited utility in ASI, it is a key dynamic stabilizer for PSI.[13] The subscapularis, along with the infraspinatus and teres minor, counterbalances the superior directed force of the deltoid. Furthermore, strengthening these muscles compresses the humeral head, maintaining stability within the glenoid.

There are poor prognostic indicators for conservative management, as seen with ASI. A painful jerk test is notable for poor response to rehabilitation and will likely need surgical intervention.[16] More consistent with traumatic etiology, surgical stabilization with an osseous repair is recommended for glenoid or humeral bone loss. Furthermore, a positive Kim test or evidence of labral or other soft-tissue pathology may experience unsatisfactory results with conservative management.[15]

Symptom persistence despite appropriate rehabilitation is an indication of surgical intervention. Although it is more common in individuals with traumatic etiology, soft-tissue defects can be present without trauma and is a common cause of conservative management failure. However, without evidence of significant bone loss, aggressive rehabilitation is the preferred primary option.

MULTIDIRECTIONAL INSTABILITY REHABILITATION

First-line treatment of MDI is rehabilitation.[20,21,41] These patients typically present with a subtle onset of pain due to the microtrauma endured from repetitive movements or hyperlaxity.

Scapular dyskinesia is a widely recognized manifestation of MDI denoted by a drooping scapula.[37] Of the limited protocols available, scapular kinematics is a heavy focus.[42,43] Strengthening the rotator cuff and periscapular muscles is the mainstay of treatment. The goal of therapy is to improve humeral head centering with the glenoid through compressional forces conducted by the rotator cuff and proprioceptive control of the scapular stabilizers.[21] A two-part series developed by Watson and colleagues[42,43] offers a detailed 6-stage rehabilitation program for MDI.

MDI rehabilitation has shown immediate subjective improvement in atraumatic instability.[44,45] Long-term outcomes are less definitive, but unsuccessful rehabilitation is more predictive in young, athletic patients or those with traumatic etiology.[44,46] Though rehabilitation efforts have shown improvements in functional status, strength, and scapular positioning,[45] not all patients respond favorably.

Before consideration of surgical intervention, a patient generally needs to have failed at least 6 months of extensive therapy. A psychological component has a role in MDI. It is imperative to distinguish between patients that voluntarily dislocate the GHJ from those that avoid positional instability despite the ability to reproduce dislocation. Voluntary dislocation has a poor prognosis with surgical treatment, whereas patients who avoid positional instability have a favorable response to operative stabilization.[21] MDI presents challenging scenarios that require collaborative decision-making. Surgical treatment has progressed substantially in recent years, and it is a viable option for those with debilitating symptoms despite rehabilitation.

RETURN TO PLAY FOR ATHLETES

In athletes, RTP is naturally the most influential consideration in determining how to proceed with management. Despite the acceptable RTP percentages following in-season rehabilitation, evidence suggests surgical intervention results in a lower recurrence rate and more successful RTP without recurrence.[27,47] In the National Football League (NFL), surgical stabilization after an instability event reduces the recurrence rate.[48] Nonetheless, an athlete may forego surgical stabilization and RTP. Therefore, it is imperative to fully educate the athlete on potential risks and complications for both surgical and nonsurgical management.

Athletes need to prove they can perform sport-specific requirements before returning. Therefore, rehabilitation focuses on activities that comprise these movements. Fatigue is a significant contributor to primary and recurrent injury. In addition to sport-specific actions, endurance is essential to meet RTP criteria. When strength, motion, endurance, and sport-specific tasks are performed equivalent to the contralateral side without pain or apprehension, an athlete may receive clearance for RTP by medical personnel.[27]

Subjective considerations are essential, as everyone progresses at different rates, but generally, RTP has a quick turnaround for the mid-season athlete and can be achieved within 3 weeks.[29,49] Dislocation, compared with subluxation, will typically increase the amount of time for RTP.[48,50] Collision sports should also be considered as this significantly increases the risk for recurrence. Failure to RTP, instability after RTP, or even successful RTP patients should be reevaluated following the season to discuss the best steps forward.

ADJUNCTIVE TREATMENT DURING REHABILITATION

Adjunctive treatment options may contribute toward therapeutic efforts during rehabilitation. If elected, these modalities are in conjunction with the previous rehabilitation protocol.

Patients may benefit from using cryotherapy in the immediate post-injury phase by decreasing inflammation.[49] Heating before, icing after, and using ultrasound during physical therapy can reduce pain and muscle spasms.

Extra support can be gained through therapeutic tape or bracing. Though there is a lack of evidence supporting functional improvement or decreased risk of recurrence, there is subjective improvement in security, posturing, and proprioception.[37] Bracing, especially in athletes, is a viable option for improvement and confidence while restricting provocative movements.[27,49] However, athletes may decline to brace as they tend to be restrictive.

Posterior shoulder stiffness is a perpetuating factor for abnormal shoulder kinematics in ASI.[27] Posterior capsular and anterior shoulder stiffness contribute similarly to PSI.[13] Joint mobilization stretches to improve flexibility are important adjunctive exercises to regain full mobility.[39]

SHOULDER INSTABILITY POSTOPERATIVE REHABILITATION PROTOCOL

Postoperative rehabilitation maintains the same primary objective as nonoperative management with one fundamental exception: protect the repair. Implementing a rehabilitation program following shoulder stabilization is essential to restore optimum functionality.

The Multicenter Orthopedic Outcomes Network (MOON) shoulder instability study began in 2012 to identify outcome predictors following shoulder stabilization.[51] The MOON shoulder instability postoperative rehabilitation protocol is based on their findings and clinical expertise (Table 3).[52]

SUMMARY

The shoulder is the most mobile joint in the body. However, the wide ROM through minimal articulation increases the risk for instability. A complex network of static and dynamic stabilizers maintains proper shoulder alignment and overall function. Injury of the GHJ stabilizers is a common feature of subluxation, dislocation, and repetitive microtrauma.

Owing to the complexity of the shoulder, a detailed history and physical examination are essential. Plain film radiographs and MRI further evaluate bony and soft-tissue damage. CT is used to quantify the degree of bone loss.

ASI is the predominant form of instability. It is usually a result of trauma in an abducted, flexed, and externally rotated arm. Identification of structural deficits,

Table 3
Multicenter Orthopedic Outcomes Network shoulder stabilization rehabilitation protocol

	Timeline	Stage	Goal	Activity	Anterior Stabilization Limitations	Posterior Stabilization Limitations
Phase I	0–2 wk	Protection	Protect repair; reduce pain and inflammation	Immobilization (sling with ABD pillow) ROM—elbow, wrist	No shoulder ROM	No shoulder ROM
Phase II	2–6 wk	ROM	Pain free and symmetric motion bilaterally		No combined ABD and ER	No combined ABD and IR
	2–4 wk	PROM/AAROM		Submaximal isometrics	90° FF, ER-S to neutral; No isometric IR/ER	90° FF; No combined ABD and IR
	4–6 wk	PROM/AAROM		Submaximal isometrics	120° FF, 90° ABD, 20° ER-S	120° FF, 90° ABD; No isometric ER
				Scapular protraction/ retraction		
Phase III	6–12 wk	Strength	Full active ROM, improve muscular strength	Discontinue sling	No anterior glides	No posterior glides
	6–8 wk	AROM		Resisted isometrics	No resisted IR	No resisted ER/IR
	8–10 wk	Strength		Theraband resistance		30° IR-S, 45° IR with 30 ABD
	10–12 wk	Strength		Theraband resistance		No IR limitations
Phase IV	12–18 wk	Sport specific	Improve power and endurance	Advanced strength/power	No limitations	No limitations
Phase V	18–24 wk	Return to play	Pass functional tests; return to sport	Functional test assessment	No limitations	No limitations

Abbreviations: AAROM, assisted active ROM; ABD, abduction; AROM, active ROM; ER, external rotation; ER-S, ER-side; FF, forward flexion; IR, internal rotation; IR-S, IR-side; PROM, passive ROM; ROM, range of motion.

including Bankart and Hill-Sachs lesions, is essential in determining the risk for recurrent instability and the role of surgical intervention.

PSI often presents with insidious onset of pain rather than instability. Repetitive microtrauma to the thin posterior band of the IGHL appears to require less force for disruption and subsequent PSI. Patients with an atraumatic etiology are typically managed conservatively. Surgical stabilization is recommended for glenoid or humeral bone loss with traumatic injuries.

MDI is symptomatic laxity in more than one plane of motion. MDI can occur in the setting of connective tissue disorders, a single traumatic event, or repetitive microtrauma. Overhead activities can result in microtrauma to the shoulder stabilizers and consequential incompetence. First-line treatment of MDI is rehabilitation. A patient that has failed at least 6 months of therapy should undergo surgical evaluation. Voluntary dislocation has a poor prognosis with surgical treatment and should be considered a last resort. Surgery is a viable option for those with debilitating symptoms despite rehabilitation or evidence of a patulous inferior capsule.

The primary goal of rehabilitation is to restore pain-free mobility, strength, and functioning. Brief immobilization followed by early passive motion is encouraged to further aid healing and pain control. Dynamic GHJ stability through gentle isometrics and rhythmic closed kinetic chain exercises restore proprioceptive control. After 4 to 6 weeks, full ROM and strengthening exercises are implemented. Rotator cuff and periscapular muscle strengthening exercises follow. Resistance and endurance exercises can be intensified as the patient progresses.

Postoperative rehabilitation maintains the same primary objective as nonoperative management while protecting the repair. After shoulder stabilization surgery, the patient is kept in a sling for at least 6 weeks. Passive ROM (PROM) and assisted active ROM (AAROM) exercises are initiated during this time. Active ROM (AROM) is started around 6 weeks and is expected to be restored at 8 weeks. Focus is shifted to mobility maintenance and strengthening with resisted isometrics and TheraBand exercises through week 12. Advanced strengthening and power exercises are performed during week 12. At this time, athletes can perform sport-specific activities. Finally, functional testing for RTP can be considered after 18 weeks.

CLINICS CARE POINTS

- The glenohumeral joint is the most dislocated joint in the body.
- Excessive retroversion of the glenoid increases the susceptibility to recurrent posterior instability.
- Conservative management in a population less than 26 years of age leads to high failure rates.
- Arthroscopic management of first-time shoulder dislocation results in a lower recurrence rate and a significantly higher rate of return to play (RTP)
- Subjective function and surgery success rates for isolated Bankart repair are satisfactory.
- Glenoid and humeral defects either enlarge or develop at a significantly higher rate with recurrent instability.
- A painful jerk test and a positive Kim test have a poor response to rehabilitation.
- Immobilization does not decrease the risk for recurrence.
- Immobilization in external rotation does not provide substantial benefit.

- Multidirectional instability rehabilitation has immediate subjective improvement in atraumatic instability.
- Rehabilitation improves functional status, strength, and scapular positioning.
- Dislocation, compared with subluxation, increases the amount of time for RTP.
- Collision sports significantly increase the risk for recurrence.

DISCLOSURE

The authors have nothing to disclose.

ACKNOWLEDGMENTS

The authors thank and acknowledge Dave Daniels MD, and Kevin Shinsako PA-C, for their assistance with photographs for this article.

REFERENCES

1. Apostolakos JM, Wright-Chisem J, Gulotta LV, et al. Anterior glenohumeral instability: current review with technical pearls and pitfalls of arthroscopic soft-tissue stabilization. World J Orthopedics 2021;12(1):1–13.
2. Abrams R, Akbarnia H. Shoulder dislocations overview. Treasure Island (FL): StatPearls; 2022. StatPearls Publishing Copyright © 2022, StatPearls Publishing LLC.
3. Cameron KL, Mauntel TC, Owens BD. The epidemiology of glenohumeral joint instability: incidence, burden, and long-term consequences. Sports Med Arthrosc Rev 2017;25(3):144–9.
4. Owens BD, Agel J, Mountcastle SB, et al. Incidence of glenohumeral instability in collegiate athletics. Am J Sports Med 2009;37(9):1750–4 [published Online First: 20090625].
5. DeFroda SF, Donnelly JC, Mulcahey MK, et al. Shoulder instability in women compared with men: epidemiology, pathophysiology, and special considerations. JBJS Rev 2019;7(9):e10.
6. Burkhart SS, De Beer JF. Traumatic glenohumeral bone defects and their relationship to failure of arthroscopic Bankart repairs: significance of the inverted-pear glenoid and the humeral engaging Hill-Sachs lesion. Arthroscopy 2000;16(7): 677–94.
7. Chang LR, Anand P, Varacallo M. Anatomy, shoulder and upper limb, glenohumeral joint. Treasure Island (FL): StatPearls; 2022. StatPearls Publishing Copyright © 2022, StatPearls Publishing LLC.
8. Kelkar R, Wang VM, Flatow EL, et al. Glenohumeral mechanics: a study of articular geometry, contact, and kinematics. J Shoulder Elbow Surg 2001;10(1): 73–84.
9. Vezeridis PS, Ishmael CR, Jones KJ, et al. Glenohumeral dislocation arthropathy: etiology, diagnosis, and management. J Am Acad Orthop Surg 2019;27(7): 227–35.
10. Frank RM, Romeo AA. Arthroscopic soft tissue reconstruction in anterior shoulder instability. Orthopade 2018;47(2):121–8.
11. Nolte PC, Elrick BP, Bernholt DL, et al. The bony Bankart: clinical and technical considerations. Sports Med Arthrosc Rev 2020;28(4):146–52.

12. Bottoni CR, Franks BR, Moore JH, et al. Operative stabilization of posterior shoulder instability. Am J Sports Med 2005;33(7):996–1002 [published Online First: 20050511].

13. Goldenberg BT, Goldsten P, Lacheta L, et al. Rehabilitation following posterior shoulder stabilization. Int J Sports Phys Ther 2021;16(3):930–40 [published Online First: 20210601].

14. McMahon PJ, Tibone JE, Cawley PW, et al. The anterior band of the inferior glenohumeral ligament: biomechanical properties from tensile testing in the position of apprehension. J Shoulder Elbow Surg 1998;7(5):467–71.

15. Frank RM, Romeo AA, Provencher MT. Posterior glenohumeral instability: evidence-based treatment. J Am Acad Orthop Surg 2017;25(9):610–23.

16. Brelin A, Dickens JF. Posterior shoulder instability. Sports Med Arthrosc Rev 2017;25(3):136–43. https://doi.org/10.1097/jsa.0000000000000160.

17. Provencher MT, Midtgaard KS, Owens BD, et al. Diagnosis and management of traumatic anterior shoulder instability. J Am Acad Orthop Surg 2021;29(2): e51–61.

18. Gottschalk MB, Ghasem A, Todd D, et al. Posterior shoulder instability: does glenoid retroversion predict recurrence and contralateral instability? Arthroscopy 2015;31(3):488–93 [published Online First: 20141210].

19. Owens BD, Campbell SE, Cameron KL. Risk factors for posterior shoulder instability in young athletes. Am J Sports Med 2013;41(11):2645–9 [published Online First: 20130827].

20. Best MJ, Tanaka MJ. Multidirectional instability of the shoulder: treatment options and considerations. Sports Med Arthrosc Rev 2018;26(3):113–9.

21. Gaskill TR, Taylor DC, Millett PJ. Management of multidirectional instability of the shoulder. J Am Acad Orthop Surg 2011;19(12):758–67.

22. Broida SE, Sweeney AP, Gottschalk MB, et al. Management of shoulder instability in hypermobility-type Ehlers-Danlos syndrome. JSES Rev Rep Tech 2021;1(3): 155–64.

23. Lizzio VA, Meta F, Fidai M, et al. Clinical evaluation and physical exam findings in patients with anterior shoulder instability. Curr Rev Musculoskelet Med 2017; 10(4):434–41.

24. Haley CCA. History and physical examination for shoulder instability. Sports Med Arthrosc Rev 2017;25(3):150–5.

25. Wolf JM, Cameron KL, Owens BD. Impact of joint laxity and hypermobility on the musculoskeletal system. J Am Acad Orthop Surg 2011;19(8):463–71.

26. De Filippo M, Schirò S, Sarohia D, et al. Imaging of shoulder instability. Skeletal Radiol 2020;49(10):1505–23 [published Online First: 20200523].

27. Wolf BR, Tranovich MA, Marcussen B, et al. Team approach: treatment of shoulder instability in athletes. JBJS Rev 2021;9(11) [published Online First: 20211110].

28. Bottoni CR, Wilckens JH, DeBerardino TM, et al. A prospective, randomized evaluation of arthroscopic stabilization versus nonoperative treatment in patients with acute, traumatic, first-time shoulder dislocations. Am J Sports Med 2002;30(4): 576–80.

29. Dickens JF, Owens BD, Cameron KL, et al. Return to play and recurrent instability after in-season anterior shoulder instability: a prospective multicenter study. Am J Sports Med 2014;42(12):2842–50 [published Online First: 20141105].

30. Gigis I, Heikenfeld R, Kapinas A, et al. Arthroscopic versus conservative treatment of first anterior dislocation of the shoulder in adolescents. J Pediatr Orthop 2014;34(4):421–5.

31. De Carli A, Vadalà AP, Lanzetti R, et al. Early surgical treatment of first-time anterior glenohumeral dislocation in a young, active population is superior to conservative management at long-term follow-up. Int Orthop 2019;43(12):2799–805 [published Online First: 20190807].

32. Hurley ET, Manjunath AK, Bloom DA, et al. Arthroscopic Bankart repair versus conservative management for first-time traumatic anterior shoulder instability: a systematic review and meta-analysis. Arthroscopy 2020;36(9):2526–32 [published Online First: 20200508].

33. Brophy RH, Marx RG. The treatment of traumatic anterior instability of the shoulder: nonoperative and surgical treatment. Arthroscopy 2009;25(3):298–304.

34. Owens BD, DeBerardino TM, Nelson BJ, et al. Long-term follow-up of acute arthroscopic Bankart repair for initial anterior shoulder dislocations in young athletes. Am J Sports Med 2009;37(4):669–73 [published Online First: 20090213].

35. Nakagawa S, Iuchi R, Hanai H, et al. The development process of bipolar bone defects from primary to recurrent instability in shoulders with traumatic anterior instability. Am J Sports Med 2019;47(3):695–703 [published Online First: 20190123].

36. Ma R, Brimmo OA, Li X, et al. Current concepts in rehabilitation for traumatic anterior shoulder instability. Curr Rev Musculoskelet Med 2017;10(4):499–506.

37. Jaggi A, Alexander S. Rehabilitation for shoulder instability – current approaches. Open Orthopaedics J 2017;11(1):957–71.

38. Kane P, Bifano SM, Dodson CC, et al. Approach to the treatment of primary anterior shoulder dislocation: a review. Phys Sportsmed 2015;43(1):54–64 [published Online First: 20150106].

39. Cools AM, Borms D, Castelein B, et al. Evidence-based rehabilitation of athletes with glenohumeral instability. Knee Surg Sports Traumatol Arthrosc 2016;24(2):382–9 [published Online First: 20151224].

40. Cools AM, Struyf F, De Mey K, et al. Rehabilitation of scapular dyskinesis: from the office worker to the elite overhead athlete. Br J Sports Med 2014;48(8):692–7 [published Online First: 20130518].

41. Coyner KJ, Arciero RA. Shoulder instability: anterior, posterior, multidirectional, arthroscopic versus open, bone block procedures. Sports Med Arthrosc Rev 2018;26(4):168–70.

42. Watson L, Warby S, Balster S, et al. The treatment of multidirectional instability of the shoulder with a rehabilitation programme: Part 2. Shoulder Elbow 2017;9(1):46–53 [published Online First: 20160708].

43. Watson L, Warby S, Balster S, et al. The treatment of multidirectional instability of the shoulder with a rehabilitation program: part 1. Shoulder Elbow 2016;8(4):271–8 [published Online First: 20160601].

44. Burkhead WZ Jr, Rockwood CA Jr. Treatment of instability of the shoulder with an exercise program. J Bone Joint Surg Am 1992;74(6):890–6.

45. Watson L, Balster S, Lenssen R, et al. The effects of a conservative rehabilitation program for multidirectional instability of the shoulder. J Shoulder Elbow Surg 2018;27(1):104–11 [published Online First: 20170922].

46. Misamore GW, Sallay PI, Didelot W. A longitudinal study of patients with multidirectional instability of the shoulder with seven- to ten-year follow-up. J Shoulder Elbow Surg 2005;14(5):466–70.

47. Dickens JF, Rue JP, Cameron KL, et al. Successful return to sport after arthroscopic shoulder stabilization versus nonoperative management in contact athletes with anterior shoulder instability: a prospective multicenter study. Am J Sports Med 2017;45(11):2540–6 [published Online First: 20170628].

48. Okoroha KR, Taylor KA, Marshall NE, et al. Return to play after shoulder instability in National Football League athletes. J Shoulder Elbow Surg 2018;27(1):17–22 [published Online First: 20170920].
49. Owens BD, Dickens JF, Kilcoyne KG, et al. Management of mid-season traumatic anterior shoulder instability in athletes. J Am Acad Orthop Surg 2012;20(8): 518–26.
50. Lu Y, Okoroha KR, Patel BH, et al. Return to play and performance after shoulder instability in National Basketball Association athletes. J Shoulder Elbow Surg 2020;29(1):50–7 [published Online First: 20190819].
51. Kraeutler MJ, McCarty EC, Belk JW, et al. Descriptive epidemiology of the MOON shoulder instability cohort. Am J Sports Med 2018;46(5):1064–9.
52. Hettrich CM, Wolf BR. MOON shoulder instability anterior stabilization therapy protocol. MOON Shoulder Group, University of Iowa; 2012.

Rehabilitation after Shoulder Instability Surgery

Jeffrey R. Hill, MD[a], John Motley, PT, ATC, CSCS[b], Jay D. Keener, MD, PT[a],*

KEYWORDS

- Rehabilitation • Shoulder instability • Glenohumeral instability
- Traumatic anterior instability • Multidirectional instability
- Neuromuscular electrical stimulation

INTRODUCTION
Anatomy

The glenohumeral articulation is largely devoid of static constraints. The large radius of curvature of the glenoid fossa creates a shallow articulation for the humeral head, allowing complex motions that include rotation and translation in multiple planes. This predisposes the glenohumeral joint to instability, particularly with acute or repetitive trauma in vulnerable positions or in the presence of structural or functional abnormalities of the dynamic stabilizers.

Furthermore, several authors have demonstrated that patients with glenohumeral instability exhibit scapular morphology that is distinctly different from normal controls. The glenoid morphology of these patients may include an increased height-width ratio, flatter radius of curvature in the anterior–posterior and superior–inferior planes, and relative anterior tilt.[1–3] The position of the coracoid process is also abnormal—often with decreased length and a more superior and medial position.[3] This may place the conjoint tendon—an important dynamic stabilizer[4]—in a disadvantageous position, and explain why an increasing coracohumeral distance has been significantly associated with risk of anterior instability.[2]

Epidemiology

Glenohumeral instability can occur in any direction and presents across a broad spectrum including traumatic dislocations, repetitive microinstability events or subluxations, and global joint laxity. The development of pain, functional decline, and articular pathologic condition is a multifaceted process that is influenced by the underlying bony morphology, biology of the surrounding soft tissue structures, dynamic coordination of the periscapular musculature, and patient factors such as age, activity level, and associated injuries. This article will focus on the younger, active patient

a Department of Orthopedic Surgery, Washington University, 660 S Euclid Avenue, CB 8233, St. Louis, MO 63110, USA; b Barnes Jewish West County Hospital, 12634 Olive Boulevard, Creve Couer, MO 63141, USA
* Corresponding author.
E-mail address: keenerj@wustl.edu

Phys Med Rehabil Clin N Am 34 (2023) 409–425
https://doi.org/10.1016/j.pmr.2022.12.007
1047-9651/23/© 2022 Elsevier Inc. All rights reserved.

with instability due to deficiencies in the capsulolabral complex and dynamic stabilizers. Rehabilitation for glenohumeral instability in patients aged older than 40 to 50 years, in which a traumatic rotator cuff tear is the primary pathology, will not be discussed.

Traumatic anterior instability is the most common form of glenohumeral instability, with an estimated incidence of 1.7%.[5] These injuries occur with much higher frequency in collision and overhead athletes, accounting for up to 20% of shoulder and elbow injuries in this population.[6] Military personnel are also at risk, with reported instability rates as much as an order of magnitude greater than the general population.[7] Posterior instability is relatively rare, representing 10% to 12% of shoulder instability cases.[8–10] This typically occurs in the form of recurrent subluxations or microinstability in patients who participate in activities requiring repetitive loading in flexion, adduction, and internal rotation.[10] Traumatic posterior dislocations are uncommon and are usually due to a traumatic accident or seizure.[11] Multidirectional instability (MDI) is caused by abnormalities of the periarticular soft tissue stabilizers. This is often associated with an underlying connective tissue disorder leading to generalized hyperlaxity but can also be seen in athletes whose shoulders are subjected to repetitive heavy loads or large motion arcs such as weightlifters, gymnasts, and swimmers.[12,13] These patients may or may not have associated labral tears. Posterior-predominant MDI, in particular, can present with a significant element of scapular dyskinesia and pathologic neuromuscular activation patterns.[14]

General Principles of Rehabilitation

Animal models have shown that histologic and biomechanical labral healing may occur as early as 4 weeks postoperatively, indicating that the process likely takes at least 6 weeks in humans.[15] Peak remodeling occurs during postoperative weeks 1 through 8[16] but the complete healing process may take up to 12 weeks.[17] Osseous healing for bony Bankart repairs or bone block augmentation procedures typically occurs within 6 to 8 weeks[16,17] but complete osseous union may require 3 to 5 months.[18] If a subscapularis tenotomy is performed as part of an open stabilization procedure, the timeline for tendon healing is generally accepted to be 6 weeks.

The core goals of shoulder rehabilitation are 3-fold.[19] During the early phases, the primary aim is to protect the healing tissues while minimizing deleterious effects of immobilization. As recovery progresses, focus shifts to restoration of functional range-of-motion (ROM), restoring dynamic joint stability, and joint proprioception. Throughout the process, reduction of pain, inflammation, and compensatory muscle activation is essential. To accomplish these goals, several key principles should be considered.[20]

- Clinically relevant glenohumeral ROM deficits should be addressed in a manner that protects the repair.
- As glenohumeral ROM improves, controlled strengthening of the core rotator cuff muscles begins.
- Attention must be paid to the entire kinetic chain, including functional contributions from the lower extremities, abdominal and lumbar spine stabilizers, and scapulothoracic articulation.
- Latter stages of rehabilitation should include exercises at low resistance and high repetition to enhance endurance in the upper extremity, closed chain exercises at low-to-moderate loads and plyometric activities. Complex, multiplanar movements that mimic the demands of the patient's desired activity are the final bridge from rehabilitation to a successful return to performance.

- Shoulder irritability should guide progression of therapy, regardless of the procedure or underlying pathologic condition. A highly irritable shoulder is indicated by high pain levels at rest, pain at night, and significant disability. In contrast, a patient with a minimally irritated shoulder will report low overall pain levels, with pain occurring only during a limited set of specific activities or movements. A staged approach to rehabilitation based on irritability has been proposed[21] but is out of the scope of this article.
- The cognitive aspect of recovery should not be ignored. Cognitive exercises may further enhance the likelihood of full return to desired function.

PATIENT EVALUATION OVERVIEW
History

On returning for follow-up visits, several topics should be discussed with the patient. To align patient and provider expectations for recovery, the timeline for rehabilitation should be emphasized early, and revisited at each subsequent encounter. Compliance with precautions, restrictions, and sling wear is essential, particularly in the early phases. Assessment of pain and shoulder irritability may be difficult in the immediate postoperative period but is important as the patient begins to progress through graduated motion and strengthening. In the later stages, assessing the patient's level of confidence in their shoulder is important. This should include reports of any obvious subluxations as well as subtle feelings of instability. When entering the final phase of recovery, it is helpful to revisit the patient's functional goals for recreation and sport as well as for their occupation.

Physical Examination

A standard postoperative examination should always include an evaluation of the surgical incision(s) and a detailed neurovascular examination. The axillary and musculocutaneous nerves are most vulnerable,[22] particularly for open procedures and those involving coracoid transfer but all terminal branches of the brachial plexus should be assessed for both motor and sensory function. Visual inspection of scapular posture is also essential because abnormal posturing may be seen after surgery due to deactivation, pain, and deconditioning of the periscapular musculature. Elbow stiffness is not uncommon because there is fear of motion and excessive sling dependence. Early identification and correction of abnormal scapular posture is a critical foundation for the entirety of the rehabilitation process. Glenohumeral ROM should also be assessed. This will vary according to the time from surgery, the direction of instability treated, whether the procedure was arthroscopic or open, and whether concomitant procedures were performed (eg, bone grafting, remplissage, subscapularis tenotomy). Finally, in later stages, the stability and laxity of the shoulder should be compared with the contralateral shoulder, specifically assessing for the presence of apprehension with provocative maneuvers, excessive external rotation with the arm at the side, presence of a sulcus sign, and hyperabduction greater than 90° (ie, Gagey test[23]).

POSTOPERATIVE REHABILITATION PROTOCOLS
Overview

Much of the orthopedic literature surrounding the topic of postoperative rehabilitation consists of studies evaluating surgical outcomes, which provide varying levels of detail regarding rehabilitation protocols. Given that traumatic anterior instability is the most common pathologic condition, it has seen the most research interest. However, there remains a paucity of high-level evidence to guide surgeons in developing a robust postoperative rehabilitation protocol. In general, 4 phases are commonly described but the specifics of each may vary depending on surgeon preference, direction and type of instability, surgical procedure performed, and patient factors and goals. Phase 1 typically encompasses the first 6 weeks and is designed to protect the surgical repair while allowing enough controlled motion to maintain articular physiology and prevent stiffness. Phase 2 represents the second 6 weeks, during which glenohumeral ROM and scapular mechanics are restored. Phase 3 spans from 3 to 6 months postoperatively, consisting of progressive strengthening and terminal stretching. Phase 4 represents the final 1 to 2 months of therapy and may overlap with phase 3, consisting of sport-specific activities with gradual progression to full performance.

Phase 1 (Weeks 0–6)

The goals of this phase are to minimize pain and inflammation while protecting the repair construct and allowing sufficient motion to prevent stiffness. This is a delicate balance—while application of controlled stress may stimulate fibroblastic differentiation and promote collagen fiber deposition, excessive micromotion can disrupt tissue regeneration at the early repair interface.[19] Other goals include correction or maintenance of appropriate scapular posture and reactivation of neuromuscular pathways. For athletes, it is also important to maintain baseline aerobic conditioning. During phase 1 the patient may perform submaximal and pain-free isometrics. Modalities such as cryotherapy and electrical stimulation may be incorporated to reduce pain and inflammation.

Immobilization typically consists of sling use for 3 to 6 weeks but consensus on the optimal duration is lacking. Accelerated protocols, most commonly used for simple cases of anterior instability, typically involve 3 weeks of immobilization.[19] Routine use of an abduction pillow is not necessary but can be helpful when more support is needed for complex repairs, or when patient compliance is a concern. Similarly, a gunslinger orthosis can be used for cases with complex or revision repairs, where the need for arm support is greater or strict immobilization is preferred. For posterior instability, immobilization in neutral or relative external rotation in reference to a standard sling position is recommended.

Scapular posture and mobilization must be a central focus during this early recovery phase. Scapular protraction and depression occurs commonly in the immediate postoperative period due to both pain and sling use (**Fig. 1**). Strengthening and stretching exercises to reposition the scapula into its proper position is critical for the success of the rehabilitation program.

Active ROM is generally initiated within the first 2 weeks to promote return of muscle activity. This should occur only in safe, prescribed arcs of motion that will not impair healing of the repaired capsule or labrum. The directions of these motions will vary based on the direction of instability and the type of repair performed but should begin within the standard cardinal planes (**Fig. 2**). For standard anterior soft tissue stabilization procedures, we recommend targets of 130° of flexion, 120° of abduction in the scapular plane, and 45° of external rotation with the arm at the side. Internal rotation behind the back and combined abduction and external rotation should be avoided. For posterior stabilization procedures, we recommend 90° of flexion, 45° of external rotation with the arm at the side, and avoidance of internal rotation or cross-body motions. If the subscapularis is tenotomized and repaired, active internal rotation should be restricted for the first 6 weeks. Passive ROM can be performed within the bounds of active ROM defined above but should not exceed these limits (generally 30–45° maximum).

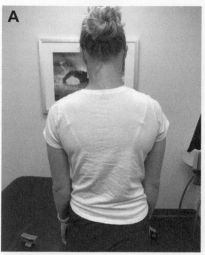 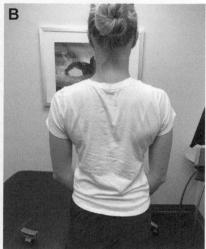

Fig. 1. Scapula posture. (*A*). Scapula protracted position. (*B*). Active scapular retraction and depression to recruit posterior scapular muscles.

Light motor recruitment can begin with submaximal isometric exercises at 3 weeks if the subscapularis was not repaired. During this phase, the patient should also work to restore and maintain their baseline aerobic capacity. A stationary or recumbent bike is the preferred option, because it does not require the upper extremities for power or stability, and does not involve impact that might compromise the repair. Patients should avoid exertion for the first 2 weeks to protect their incisions from sweat.

Phase 2 (Weeks 6–12)

The primary goals of this phase are to regain functional motion and begin restoration of dynamic stability. This should include progression of glenohumeral motion without aggressive stretching, and gradual strengthening of the rotator cuff and periscapular musculature. In many programs, immobilization is discontinued at this time. Patients who were previously immobilized in a gunslinger orthosis can either discontinue immobilization completely or can transition to a sling for 4 weeks if prolonged protection is desired.

Active and passive motion should be progressed gradually in the cardinal planes (diagonal planes will be initiated in late Phase 2 or early Phase 3) and should be performed within the following limits. For anterior stabilization: flexion and abduction in the scapular plane as tolerated, external rotation with arm at the side to 60°, internal rotation as

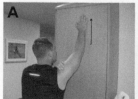 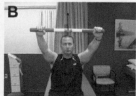 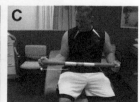

Fig. 2. Active range of motion—phases 1 and 2. Individualized motion limits are emphasized. (*A*) Wall slides with scapula stabilization. (*B*) Antigravity wand-assisted elevation. (*C*) Wand-assisted external rotation motion.

tolerated, and avoidance of combined external-rotation/abduction stretching. Anterior joint glides can facilitate external rotation motion without excessive capsular stretch (**Fig. 3**) For posterior stabilization: flexion should be limited to 130°, external rotation to tolerance both with arm at the side and in abduction, no aggressive internal rotation stretching, and cross-body motion limited to light movements only. Terminal passive ROM and capsular stretching should not begin earlier than 6 weeks—the direction and magnitude of which should be individualized based on the direction of instability and the nature of the repair procedure. If the subscapularis was repaired, passive external rotation stretching should be limited for the first 6 weeks to protect the repair, with the specific limit determined by intraoperative ROM (typically 30°–45°).

Reactivation and strengthening of the dynamic stabilizers is a core component of this phase. Similar to phase 1, attention to the scapula is essential. As scapulothoracic motion progresses, focus must remain on proper scapular posture but should now also be placed on scapular control with antigravity elevation. Progressive strengthening of the periscapular musculature and rotator cuff should occur throughout this phase, starting with isotonic exercises within the arcs of motion defined above (**Figs 4 and 5**). Electrical stimulation of the posterior cuff musculature may be incorporated into the rehabilitation program to enhance muscle fiber recruitment. Additionally, early initiation and progression of proprioceptive training is beneficial. In the early stages, closed-chain exercises will facilitate muscular cocontraction and proprioception (**Fig. 6**). In later stages, rhythmic stabilization drills can be introduced and proprioceptive neuromuscular facilitation patterns initiated.

Phase 3 (Months 3–6)

The goals of this phase are 2-fold. First, patients must regain terminal ROM to allow safe return to their prior level of performance. In concert with this, the functional strength, power, and endurance required for the patient's desired activities must also be restored.

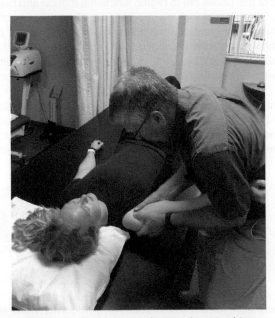

Fig. 3. Manual anterior glides to facilitate gentle capsular stretching.

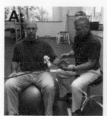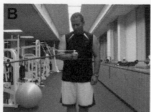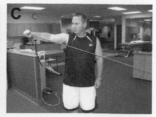

Fig. 4. Isotonic rotator cuff strengthening exercises. (*A*) Theraband external rotation isometric with rhythmic stabilization with core trunk stabilization balancing. (*B*) Theraband internal rotation. (*C*) Theraband resisted scapular plane elevation.

The goal of both active and passive motions in this phase is to restore full capsular mobility and active ROM while maintaining normal scapular mechanics. Continuing from late phase 2, motion during the early stages of phase 3 should progress from the cardinal planes to arcs across planes in order to replicate normal function. For anterior stabilization, goals include normalization of terminal flexion, abduction in the scapular plane, external rotation with arm at the side, and internal rotation.

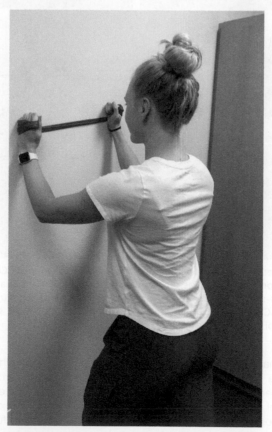

Fig. 5. Multiposition shoulder isometrics. Resisted isometric external rotation with theraband at graduated levels of elevation.

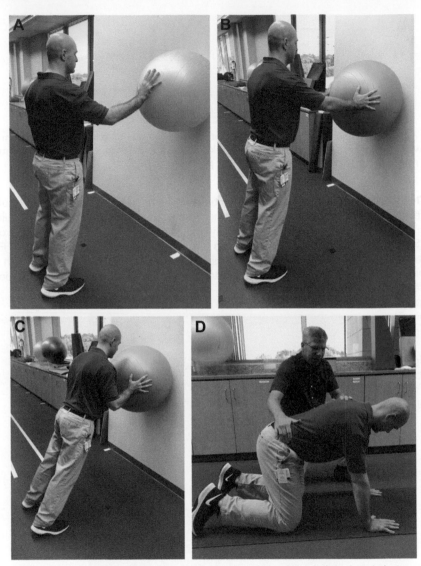

Fig. 6. Closed kinetic chain exercises. Emphasis on motor control. (*A*) Closed chain active pendulum elevation with emphasis on scapular posture. (*B*) Closed chain swiss ball push up shoulder press–starting position. (*C*) Closed chain swiss ball push up shoulder press–end position. (*D*) Closed chain quadruped shoulder compression with serratus activation with rhythmic stabilization and isometric resistance to body sway.

Combined external-rotation/abduction stretching can begin during this phase. For patients in whom a remplissage was performed, ROM in external-rotation/abduction may be decreased compared with isolated Bankart repairs.[24] These patients may require additional time and attention to maximize restoration of external rotation in this plane. For posterior stabilization, goals include restoration of full flexion as well as external and internal rotation. Isolated posterior capsule stretches can facilitate terminal motion in patients with residual posterior capsule stiffness (**Fig. 7**).

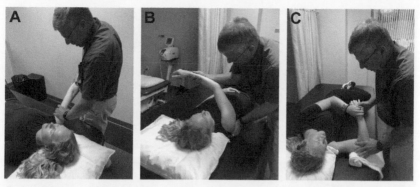

Fig. 7. Posterior capsule stretching techniques. (*A*) Manual posterior glide. (*B*) Cross-body stretching with stabilization of scapula. (*C*) Posterior capsule rotational stretch.

Strengthening during phase 3 should include advanced rotator cuff and periscapular exercises. Once the patient demonstrates adequate strength along with proper glenohumeral and scapulothoracic mechanics, they can be progressed to functional exercises (**Fig. 8**). Specific tasks should be catered to each patient based on their direction of instability, type of surgical repair, and goals for return to activity or occupation. These should include exercises involving dynamic strength and stabilization across planes, establishing neuromuscular control, at end ranges, and incorporation of the lower body to emphasize coordination throughout the entire kinetic chain (**Fig. 9**). Plyometric exercises may be incorporated to improve the patient's ability to produce and dissipate forces. Drills should initially be performed with 2 hands close to the body with progression eventually to 1 handed drills with longer lever positions away from the body.

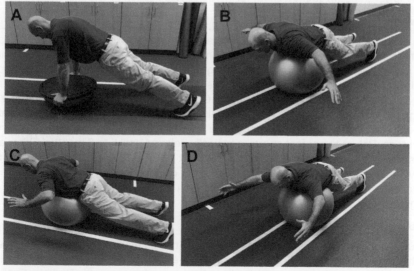

Fig. 8. Swiss ball rotator cuff and scapular stabilizer strengthening combinations. (*A*) Dynamic stabilization of body weight with scapular control. (*B*) Scapular retraction with shoulder horizontal abduction posterior deltoid ("T" position). (*C*) Scapular retraction with external rotation ("W" position). (*D*) Scapular retraction with elevation ("Y" position).

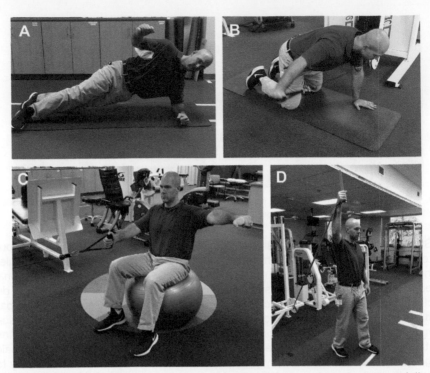

Fig. 9. Advanced strengthening techniques. Emphasized once range of motion is full and designed to simulate functional tasks. (*A*) Resisted external rotation with core muscle contraction in side plank position. (*B*) Resisted horizontal extension and scapular retraction with cable. (*C*) Resisted shoulder extension with core stabilization through trunk. (*D*) Oscillatory lower trapezius strengthening for rhythmic stabilization in terminal flexion.

Phase 4 (Month 4 and Beyond)

This phase often overlaps with the latter stages of phase 3. The primary goal of phase 4 is to facilitate a safe transition to the patient's prior level of function and performance. For patients with overhead demands, a graduated return to specific activities can begin at 4 to 6 months based on achievement of phase 3 milestones as well as the nature of the sport or occupational activity. Once the rotator cuff strength normalizes, progression to more traditional weight training is started assuming scapular control can be maintained. Throwers can begin a carefully prescribed throwing program at this stage. Return to contact sports is typically delayed until 5 to 6 months. Other athletes may return on an accelerated timeline but these decisions should be carefully individualized for each case. This requires clear communication among the surgeon, therapist, and patient, and it should be based on the underlying pathologic condition, surgical repair, and patient goals.

Return to Sport

Return to sport or activity should not be thought of as a singular milestone or event. Rather, it should occur across a continuum that encompasses return to participation, followed by return to sport, and finally return to performance.[20] "Participation" includes rehabilitation and sport-specific training, "sport" involves engaging in the desired activity at submaximal levels, and "performance" refers to unrestricted activity at preinjury levels.

Currently, there are no validated criteria for return to sport after shoulder instability procedures.[25,26] Protocols vary widely for anterior instability[25,26] and are poorly described for posterior instability and MDI. A tool modeled after that used for return-to-play following anterior cruciate ligament reconstruction—named the Shoulder Instability Return to Sport after Injury tool—has been validated[27] but not widely adopted. A 2021 survey of North American and European shoulder surgeons indicates that the most common criterion for return to sport after both arthroscopic bankart repair and latarjet is time.[28] Most surgeons allow patients to return by 4 to 6 months for arthroscopic stabilization and 3 to 4 months for latarjet. Many will delay return after arthroscopic stabilization by 1 to 3 months for collision athletes. For patients treated with either bony bankart repair or a bone augmentation procedure, we recommend computed tomography imaging to confirm bony healing before release to contact sports.

Although consensus metrics are lacking, several general principles should be considered when determining a patient's readiness to return to activity, sport, or occupation.[20] Pain should be minimal when returning to participation, and should be absent before returning to performance. Restoration of full ROM is not a requirement for return to participation but should be achieved before returning to performance—particularly for overhead and throwing athletes. Strength, power, and endurance should match either preinjury values or those of the contralateral shoulder. Kinematic motion analysis, when available, should be used to identify and correct weak links in the kinetic chain.[29] Psychologic readiness may be easily overlooked but can be crucial in helping patients overcome mental barriers related to apprehension or fear of reinjury, which may lead to pathologic compensatory movement patterns.

PATHOLOGY-SPECIFIC CONSIDERATIONS
Anterior Instability

With the use of modern techniques and implants, patients undergoing isolated arthroscopic Bankart repairs can be considered for accelerated rehabilitation programs. Level-1 evidence suggests that these programs are safe in carefully selected patients (isolated anteroinferior capsulolabral lesion, healthy labral tissue, no ligamentous laxity), with the potential for decreased postoperative pain, faster return to functional motion and activity, and improved patient satisfaction.[30] Subsequent prospective and retrospective case series have confirmed the safety of accelerated rehabilitation for active patients.[31,32] However, these programs may be less successful for contact athletes,[31] and have not been proven for overhead athletes. Accelerated rehabilitation generally involves sling use exclusively during sleep for the first 2 weeks and a gradual increase in exercises starting postoperative day 1. Patients are progressed to full ROM by week 4, with the exception of terminal external rotation.

Remplissage is an effective augment to anterior soft-tissue repairs in patients with minimal glenoid bone loss but a significant Hill-Sachs lesion (greater than 20 mm or 15%).[24,33–37] Postoperative external rotation deficits have been reported by several authors but overall seem to be transient and mild.[24,33,36] A 2022 statement from the Anterior Shoulder Instability International Consensus group states that although postoperative protocols do not need significant alteration following remplissage, potential decreases in external rotation motion should be considered during the early phases of rehabilitation.[38] Similarly, a 2021 survey of North American and European shoulder surgeons indicated that the addition of remplissage need not affect return-to-play decisions after anterior soft tissue repair.[28]

For patients undergoing an open labral repair with or without capsular shift, a more conservative approach should be taken in the early phases of rehabilitation. In most cases, a subscapularis repair must be protected in addition to the capsulolabral repair. Subscapularis healing takes a minimum of 6 weeks, extending the timeline for the advancement of passive external rotation and active internal rotation. If not appropriately protected, subscapularis deficiency can lead to inferior functional outcomes and decreased patient satisfaction.[39] Although rotational strength may recover more slowly in the early stages compared with isolated arthroscopic Bankart repairs, this typically equalizes by 1 year.[40]

Cases involving bony healing, such as bony Bankart repairs and bone augmentation procedures, can generally follow standard postoperative protocols. Due to the shorter timeframe for bony healing compared with that of the capsule and labrum, rehabilitation for these patients can be progressed more rapidly.[17] For latarjet procedures specifically, an accelerated active ROM and stretching protocol after 6 weeks may be acceptable. However, criteria and specifications of acceleration are highly variable between institutions and providers.[17] Although many surgeons are comfortable with patients returning to activity without radiographic evidence of bony union,[28] we recommend consideration of computed tomography imaging before return to contact sports.

Posterior Instability

Procedures performed for posterior instability may include arthroscopic posterior labral repair, posterior capsular shift, posterior bone block augmentation, and subscapularis or lesser tuberosity advancement. Given the lower incidence, broad spectrum of pathologic condition, and varied surgical techniques, postoperative rehabilitation protocols vary widely, with minimal high-quality evidence to guide surgeons. Currently, the literature is limited to descriptions of protocols included in the methods of cohort and case-control studies designed to evaluate surgical outcomes.[9] In contrast to anterior instability, rehabilitation need not differ significantly between arthroscopic and open repairs, given that open posterior procedures do not require takedown of the posterior rotator cuff tendons. Postoperative protocols should be tailored to each patient based on the procedure performed and their recovery goals[41] but general principles can be applied to most cases. Immobilization should maintain abduction and neutral to slight external rotation for a duration of 3 to 6 weeks.[9] A similar 4-phase framework can be applied; however, the time for complete recovery may be prolonged relative to anterior instability cases. Return to sport or demanding physical labor may take up to 8 months and is less predictable—particularly for throwing athletes, who may require especially intensive rehabilitation[9,42,43].

Multidirectional Instability

Procedures for MDI typically involve open capsular work with shifts or plications tailored to the patient's predominant insufficiency. These may also be combined with closure of the rotator interval and biceps suspension techniques. The optimal postoperative rehabilitation protocol is unclear but, in general, milestones along the 4-phase framework should be more conservative due to the higher risk of recurrent instability in these patients.[12] Specifically, a longer period of immobilization should be considered, along with slower progression of ROM in all planes. In comparison to capsular shifts for anterior instability, those for MDI may involve a greater portion of the inferior capsule, and therefore limitations on forward elevation may be prudent in the early phases.[12] Careful attention must also be directed to addressing scapular mechanics and motor control of the periscapular stabilizers.[44,45]

ADJUNCTS AND FUTURE DIRECTIONS
Neuromuscular Electrical Stimulation

Pathologic muscular activation patterns are known to contribute to shoulder insta-bility.[46] Although functional shoulder instability occurs most commonly in the posterior direction, anterior and multidirectional patterns have also been described.[14] Neuro-muscular electrical stimulation (NMES) applied to the scapular stabilizers (rhomboids and inferior trapezius) as well as the shoulder external rotators (infraspinatus, teres minor, posterior deltoid) can provide effective and durable treatment of patients with recalcitrant instability, including those who have failed prior surgical intervention.[47,48] Incorporation of NMES into postoperative rehabilitation may be most helpful for pa-tients with severely pathologic scapulothoracic and glenohumeral kinematics—partic-ularly those with posterior instability or MDI. However, some advocate utilization of electrical stimulation for all patients when initiating light strengthening in the early stages of phase 2 rehabilitation.[19]

Home Rehabilitation Programs

In recent years, interest in home-based rehabilitation programs has grown. As the driver behind the management of shoulder disorders shifts toward value-based care, cost-efficient treatment pathways are being explored.[49,50] Home therapy pro-grams may align with these goals by decreasing cost and minimizing patient burden. One randomized clinical trial has compared home rehabilitation to supervised therapy following arthroscopic Bankart repair.[51] Although limited by its small sample size, 6-month follow-up period, and narrow scope of pathology, this study provides evidence that home programs may be appropriate for carefully selected patients without the risk of early repair failure or inferior functional outcomes. Further research is needed to confirm and expand on these findings. The efficacy of home programs may be further enhanced by the concurrent increase in application of wearable technologies to post-operative monitoring following orthopedic procedures. Although this has been described for lower extremity procedures such as total knee arthroplasty,[52] data for the shoulder is limited and may be more challenging to validate given the complexity of tracking scapulothoraic and glenohumeral motion[53].

CLINICS CARE POINTS

- General principles that guide safe and successful rehabilitation after shoulder instability surgery include the following:
  - Careful protection of repair in early stages (first 2 months)
  - Early attention to scapular posture and mobilization
  - Controlled restoration of glenohumeral motion—first in the cardinal planes, progressing to movements across planes
  - Reactivation of joint proprioception
  - Progression from isometric to isotonic strengthening, followed by resistance training and sport-specific activities
  - Advancement at all stages guided by shoulder irritability
  - Consider incorporating cognitive exercises to maximize confidence and optimize performance
- Return to sport is not a singular event but rather a continuum without consensus metrics
  - Participation is the first step, encompassing rehabilitation and sport-specific training
  - Sport follows, with the initiation of the desired activity at submaximal levels
  - Performance is the final step, characterized by unrestricted activity at preinjury levels
- Anterior instability

- ○ Carefully selected patients with straightforward repairs and who are not returning to contact or overhead sports can be considered for accelerated programs
- ○ Utilization of remplissage need not alter rehabilitation or return-to-sport protocols
- ○ If the subscapularis was repaired, a more conservative approach is necessary, particularly in the first 6 weeks
- ○ For patients with bony repair or bone augmentation, rehabilitation can progress more rapidly
  - ■ Consider advanced imaging to confirm bony union before return to play
- • Posterior instability
  - ○ Initial immobilization should maintain abduction and neutral to slight external rotation
  - ○ Return to sport may take longer and is less predictable
- • Multidirectional instability
  - ○ The optimal rehabilitation regimen remains unclear—protocols should be individualized to each unique case
  - ○ Consider a longer period of immobilization and slower progression of ROM in all planes
- • In patients with severely pathologic scapulothoracic and glenohumeral kinematics, consider incorporation of early neuromuscular facilitation techniques that focus on qualitative motion.

DISCLOSURE

The authors have nothing to disclose.

REFERENCES

1. Peltz CD, Zauel R, Ramo N, et al. Differences in glenohumeral joint morphology between patients with anterior shoulder instability and healthy, uninjured volunteers. J Shoulder Elbow Surg 2015;24(7):1014–20.
2. Owens BD, Campbell SE, Cameron KL. Risk factors for anterior glenohumeral instability. Am J Sports Med 2014;42(11):2591–6.
3. Jacxsens M, Elhabian SY, Brady SE, et al. Coracoacromial morphology: a contributor to recurrent traumatic anterior glenohumeral instability? J Shoulder Elbow Surg 2019;28(7):1316–25.e1.
4. Giles JW, Boons HW, Ferreira LM, et al. The effect of the conjoined tendon of the short head of the biceps and coracobrachialis on shoulder stability and kinematics during in-vitro simulation. J Biomech 2011;44(6):1192–5.
5. Lloyd G, Day J, Lu J, et al. Postoperative rehabilitation of anterior glenohumeral joint instability surgery: a systematic review. Sports Med Arthrosc Rev 2021;29(2): 54–62.
6. Anderson MJJ, Mack CD, Herzog MM, et al. Epidemiology of shoulder instability in the national football league. Orthop J Sports Med 2021;9(5). 23259671211007744.
7. Waterman B, Owens BD, Tokish JM. Anterior shoulder instability in the military athlete. Sports Health 2016;8(6):514–9.
8. Brelin A, Dickens JF. Posterior shoulder instability. Sports Med Arthrosc Rev 2017;25(3):136–43.
9. Koczan B, Stryder B, Mitchell C. Postoperative Rehabilitation of Posterior Glenohumeral Joint Instability Surgery: A Systematic Review. Sports Med Arthrosc Rev 2021;29(2):110–8.
10. Robinson CM, Aderinto J. Recurrent posterior shoulder instability. J Bone Joint Surg Am 2005;87(4):883–92.

11. Robinson CM, Seah M, Akhtar MA. The epidemiology, risk of recurrence, and functional outcome after an acute traumatic posterior dislocation of the shoulder. J Bone Joint Surg Am 2011;93(17):1605–13.

12. Ayoub CC, Berardino K, Tsou HJ, et al. Postoperative rehabilitation of multidirectional instability surgery: a systematic review. Sports Med Arthrosc Rev 2021; 29(2):88–93.

13. Best MJ, Tanaka MJ. Multidirectional instability of the shoulder: treatment options and considerations. Sports Med Arthrosc Rev 2018;26(3):113–9.

14. Moroder P, Danzinger V, Maziak N, et al. Characteristics of functional shoulder instability. J Shoulder Elbow Surg 2020;29(1):68–78.

15. Abe H, Itoi E, Yamamoto N, et al. Healing processes of the glenoid labral lesion in a rabbit model of shoulder dislocation. Tohoku J Exp Med 2012;228(2):103–8.

16. Blackburn TA, Guido JA. Rehabilitation after Ligamentous and Labral Surgery of the Shoulder: Guiding Concepts. J Athl Train 2000;35(3):373–81.

17. Beletsky A, Cancienne JM, Manderle BJ, et al. A comparison of physical therapy protocols between open latarjet coracoid transfer and arthroscopic bankart repair. Sports Health 2020;12(2):124–31.

18. Nakagawa S, Ozaki R, Take Y, et al. Bone fragment union and remodeling after arthroscopic bony bankart repair for traumatic anterior shoulder instability with a glenoid defect: influence on postoperative recurrence of instability. Am J Sports Med 2015;43(6):1438–47.

19. Ma R, Brimmo OA, Li X, et al. Current concepts in rehabilitation for traumatic anterior shoulder instability. Curr Rev Musculoskelet Med 2017;10(4):499–506.

20. Schwank A, Blazey P, Asker M, et al. 2022 Bern consensus statement on shoulder injury prevention, rehabilitation, and return to sport for athletes at all participation levels. J Orthop Sports Phys Ther 2022;52(1):11–28.

21. McClure PW, Michener LA. Staged approach for rehabilitation classification: shoulder disorders (star-shoulder). Phys Ther 2015;95(5):791–800.

22. Delaney RA, Freehill MT, Janfaza DR, et al. 2014 Neer Award Paper: neuromonitoring the Latarjet procedure. J Shoulder Elbow Surg 2014;23(10):1473–80.

23. Balg F, Boileau P. The instability severity index score. A simple pre-operative score to select patients for arthroscopic or open shoulder stabilisation. J Bone Joint Surg Br 2007;89(11):1470–7.

24. MacDonald P, McRae S, Old J, et al. Arthroscopic Bankart repair with and without arthroscopic infraspinatus remplissage in anterior shoulder instability with a Hill-Sachs defect: a randomized controlled trial. J Shoulder Elbow Surg 2021;30(6): 1288–98.

25. Hurley ET, Montgomery C, Jamal MS, et al. Return to play after the latarjet procedure for anterior shoulder instability: a systematic review. Am J Sports Med 2019;47(12):3002–8.

26. Ciccotti MC, Syed U, Hoffman R, et al. Return to play criteria following surgical stabilization for traumatic anterior shoulder instability: a systematic review. Arthroscopy 2018;34(3):903–13.

27. Gerometta A, Klouche S, Herman S, et al. The Shoulder Instability-Return to Sport after Injury (SIRSI): a valid and reproducible scale to quantify psychological readiness to return to sport after traumatic shoulder instability. Knee Surg Sports Traumatol Arthrosc 2018;26(1):203–11.

28. Hurley ET, Matache BA, Colasanti CA, et al. Return to play criteria among shoulder surgeons following shoulder stabilization. J Shoulder Elbow Surg 2021;30(6): e317–21.

29. Chalmers PN, Wimmer MA, Verma NN, et al. The Relationship Between Pitching Mechanics and Injury: A Review of Current Concepts. Sports Health 2017;9(3): 216–21.

30. Kim SH, Ha KI, Jung MW, et al. Accelerated rehabilitation after arthroscopic Bankart repair for selected cases: a prospective randomized clinical study. Arthroscopy 2003;19(7):722–31.

31. Law BKY, Yung PSH, Ho EPY, et al. The surgical outcome of immediate arthroscopic Bankart repair for first time anterior shoulder dislocation in young active patients. Knee Surg Sports Traumatol Arthrosc 2008;16(2):188–93.

32. Gibson J, Kerss J, Morgan C, et al. Accelerated rehabilitation after arthroscopic Bankart repair in professional footballers. Shoulder & Elbow 2016;8(4):279–86.

33. Brilakis E, Avramidis G, Malahias MA, et al. Long-term outcome of arthroscopic remplissage in addition to the classic Bankart repair for the management of recurrent anterior shoulder instability with engaging Hill-Sachs lesions. Knee Surg Sports Traumatol Arthrosc 2019;27(1):305–13.

34. Buza JA, Iyengar JJ, Anakwenze OA, et al. Arthroscopic Hill-Sachs remplissage: a systematic review. J Bone Joint Surg Am 2014;96(7):549–55.

35. Zhu YM, Lu Y, Zhang J, et al. Arthroscopic Bankart repair combined with remplissage technique for the treatment of anterior shoulder instability with engaging Hill-Sachs lesion: a report of 49 cases with a minimum 2-year follow-up. Am J Sports Med 2011;39(8):1640–7.

36. Lazarides AL, Duchman KR, Ledbetter L, et al. Arthroscopic Remplissage for Anterior Shoulder Instability: A Systematic Review of Clinical and Biomechanical Studies. Arthroscopy 2019;35(2):617–28.

37. Cho NS, Yoo JH, Juh HS, et al. Anterior shoulder instability with engaging Hill-Sachs defects: a comparison of arthroscopic Bankart repair with and without posterior capsulodesis. Knee Surg Sports Traumatol Arthrosc 2016;24(12):3801–8.

38. Hurley ET, Matache BA, Wong I, et al. Anterior Shoulder Instability Part II—Latarjet, Remplissage, and Glenoid Bone-Grafting—An International Consensus Statement. Arthrosc J Arthroscopic Relat Surg 2022;38(2):224–33.e6.

39. Sachs RA, Williams B, Stone ML, et al. Open Bankart repair: correlation of results with postoperative subscapularis function. Am J Sports Med 2005;33(10): 1458–62.

40. Rhee YG, Lim CT, Cho NS. Muscle strength after anterior shoulder stabilization: arthroscopic versus open Bankart repair. Am J Sports Med 2007;35(11):1859–64.

41. Abrams JS, Savoie FH, Tauro JC, et al. Recent advances in the evaluation and treatment of shoulder instability: anterior, posterior, and multidirectional. Arthroscopy 2002;18(9 Suppl 2):1–13.

42. Bradley JP, Baker CL, Kline AJ, et al. Arthroscopic capsulolabral reconstruction for posterior instability of the shoulder: a prospective study of 100 shoulders. Am J Sports Med 2006;34(7):1061–71.

43. Tibone JE, Bradley JP. The treatment of posterior subluxation in athletes. Clin Orthop Relat Res 1993;291:124–37.

44. Gaskill TR, Taylor DC, Millett PJ. Management of multidirectional instability of the shoulder. J Am Acad Orthop Surg 2011;19(12):758–67.

45. Warby SA, Ford JJ, Hahne AJ, et al. Comparison of 2 Exercise Rehabilitation Programs for Multidirectional Instability of the Glenohumeral Joint: A Randomized Controlled Trial. Am J Sports Med 2018;46(1):87–97.

46. Jaggi A, Noorani A, Malone A, et al. Muscle activation patterns in patients with recurrent shoulder instability. Int J Shoulder Surg 2012;6(4):101–7.

47. Moroder P, Minkus M, Böhm E, et al. Use of shoulder pacemaker for treatment of functional shoulder instability: Proof of concept. Obere Extrem 2017;12(2):103–8.
48. Moroder P, Plachel F, Van-Vliet H, et al. Shoulder-Pacemaker Treatment Concept for Posterior Positional Functional Shoulder Instability: A Prospective Clinical Trial. Am J Sports Med 2020;48(9):2097–104.
49. Polisetty TS, Colley R, Levy JC. Value Analysis of Anatomic and Reverse Shoulder Arthroplasty for Glenohumeral Osteoarthritis with an Intact Rotator Cuff. J Bone Joint Surg Am 2021;103(10):913–20.
50. Black EM, Higgins LD, Warner JJP. Value-based shoulder surgery: practicing outcomes-driven, cost-conscious care. J Shoulder Elbow Surg 2013;22(7):1000–9.
51. Ismail MM, El Shorbagy KM. Motions and functional performance after supervised physical therapy program versus home-based program after arthroscopic anterior shoulder stabilization: A randomized clinical trial. Ann Phys Rehabil Med 2014;57(6–7):353–72.
52. Small SR, Bullock GS, Khalid S, et al. Current clinical utilisation of wearable motion sensors for the assessment of outcome following knee arthroplasty: a scoping review. BMJ Open 2019;9(12):e033832.
53. Williams S, Schmidt R, Disselhorst-Klug C, et al. An upper body model for the kinematical analysis of the joint chain of the human arm. J Biomech 2006;39(13):2419–29.

Managing Scapular Dyskinesis

W. Ben Kibler, MD[a], John William Lockhart, PT, DPT[b], Robin Cromwell, PT[b],
Aaron Sciascia, PhD, ATC, PES, SMTC, FNAP[c,*]

KEYWORDS

• Scapula • Rehabilitation • Kinetic chain • Motor control

KEY POINTS

- The scapula plays significant roles in developing task-specific kinematics for optimal shoulder and arm function.
- Scapular dyskinesis, defined as an alteration of scapular position at rest or upon dynamic motion, is not a specific diagnosis or an injury by itself, but an impairment of normal kinematics, and can be observed in association with most shoulder injuries.
- Scapular dyskinesis has multiple pathoanatomical and pathophysiological causative factors, all of which can be evaluated by standard clinical testing through a step-wise evaluation process.
- It is recommended clinicians allow the examination to guide the treatment. Addressing impairments such as immobility and decreased strength may be necessary, but motor control enhancement should be considered as well.

INTRODUCTION

The scapula is an integral segment in the proximal to distal kinetic chain system that creates task-specific positions and motions for shoulder and arm function. Recent studies have produced information that more precisely characterizes normal and abnormal scapular mechanics, develops more effective methods of clinical evaluation, better categorizes the causative factors of abnormal scapular kinematics, and outlines more efficacious intervention protocols that will guide functional rehabilitation. This article provides an overview of the information and highlight clinical applications.

BACKGROUND
Scapular Function

Optimal scapular function is a key component of all shoulder and arm sports, work, and everyday activities. Normal scapular position and motion are foundational for

[a] Shoulder Center of Kentucky, Lexington Clinic, 1221 South Broadway, Lexington, KY 40504, USA; [b] Department of Physical Therapy, Lexington Clinic, 1221 South Broadway, Lexington, KY 40504, USA; [c] Institute for Clinical Outcomes and Research, Lexington Clinic, 1221 South Broadway, Lexington, KY 40504, USA
* Corresponding author.
E-mail address: ascia@lexclin.com

Phys Med Rehabil Clin N Am 34 (2023) 427–451
https://doi.org/10.1016/j.pmr.2022.12.008
1047-9651/23/© 2022 Elsevier Inc. All rights reserved.

the achievement of its roles. The overall purposes of scapular motion are to optimize the dynamic task-specific balance between scapular stability and scapular mobility.[1] Scapular stability provides a stable base for optimal activation of the scapular-based muscles, a stable fulcrum for arm function as a first-class and third-class lever, and stability against the loads and momentum of arm motion. Scapular mobility provides a dynamic socket for optimal glenohumeral (GH) joint ball and socket kinematics, creating maximal concavity/compression and dynamic GH stability throughout the whole arm motion, results in positioning the arm and hand in three-dimensional space for function, and moves the acromion for optimal arm elevation.

Scapulohumeral rhythm (SHR) is the mechanism for optimal shoulder and arm function. Efficient SHR underlies efficient arm function, whereas alterations in SHR affect effective arm function and increase injury risk. The coupled motion is a ratio between individual scapular and humeral motions during arm movement in elevation. The average ratio between scapular rotation and humeral rotation over the whole arm motion up to maximal elevation is 1:2 but will vary from 1:1 to 1:4 depending upon the phases of scapular and arm motion.

Coupled motions create all SHR and arm functions[2] There are four phases of scapular motion with arm motion. Phase 1 involves setting the scapula and occurs during 0° to 30° of arm elevation. This creates the initial placement of the scapula on the thorax to optimize further and later arm motions. The primary muscle activation for motion is the serratus anterior. The SHR ratio is 1:4.

Phase 2 involves scapular rotation and occurs during 30° to 100° of arm elevation. This results in mainly upward rotation in three-dimensional task-specific patterns. The primary muscle activation for mobilization is the serratus anterior, and for control and stabilization is the trapezius. The instant center of rotation is at the medial scapular spine. The SHR ratio is 1:1.

Phase 3 involves scapular rotation at or above 100° arm elevation. This results in mainly rotation along the long axis of clavicle. The muscle activations to produce this rotation are the serratus anterior and trapezius. The force transducers to produce this rotation are the coracoclavicular (CC) and acromioclavicular (AC) ligaments. The instant center of rotation moves along the clavicle to the AC joint. There is little SHR rotation. This phase mainly positions the scapula to act as a base for GH function.

Phase 4 is characterized by controlled dynamic scapular stability at or above 100°. The exact position is dependent upon the required tasks and demands for function. The scapula performs as a stable base for GH function, optimizing concavity/compression and muscle activation. At this level, the most effective single scapular position and motion for arm function is stabilized retraction, consisting of external rotation, posterior tilt, and upward rotation. For dynamic overhead, activities-controlled protraction is also required to respond to the eccentric activities experienced during throwing.

Scapular Dysfunction (Dyskinesis)

Most scapula-related shoulder dysfunction can be traced to the loss of control of the normal resting scapular position and dynamic scapular motion, which results in alterations in position or motion that produce a position and motion of excessive protraction.[3] The altered scapular position at rest has been described as the Scapula malposition–*Inferior* medial border prominence–coracoid pain–scapular dyskinesis (SICK) scapula.[4] Altered dynamic motion is called scapular dyskinesis (the term combines *dys* [alteration of] and *kinesis* [motion]). Scapular dyskinesis is characterized by medial or inferomedial scapular border prominence, early scapular elevation or shrugging when the arm is elevated, and rapid downward rotation when the arm is lowered.[3-5] The salient clinical manifestation of the dyskinetic scapula is protraction.

Dyskinesis represents an alteration of scapular position and/or motion that may create an impairment of the ability to achieve the scapular roles. It is not a specific injury or a musculoskeletal diagnosis. Dyskinesis may be a clinically insignificant finding, with as many as 27% of identified alterations of kinematics not associated with clinical symptoms.[6] However, it is considered clinically significant when it is identified in association with symptoms and arm dysfunction.[5,7] Whether associated with symptoms or not, protraction is an unfavorable position for almost all shoulder functions and may increase the risk for subsequent injury. If it is shown on exam in the symptomatic patient or in someone who anticipates high loads during overhead activities, one of the goals of treatment or conditioning should be regaining static and dynamic retraction capability.

Multiple causative factors have been identified that can affect the static position or dynamic motion control and result in the observation of dyskinesis. These can be grouped into alterations in anatomy (pathoanatomy) or alterations in muscle activation, flexibility, or strength (pathophysiology).

Pathoanatomical causative factors include:

- Clavicle fracture
- Scapular body, glenoid fracture
- AC joint injury
- GH joint internal derangement (labral injury, GH instability, biceps tendon injury, GH arthritis, adhesive capsulitis)
- Rotator cuff injury
- Post-traumatic scapular muscle injury
- Snapping scapula
- Neurologic injury (long thoracic nerve, spinal accessory nerve, dorsal scapular nerve, cervical radiculopathy)

Pathophysiological causative factors include:

- Soft tissue tightness (pectoralis minor, upper trapezius, latissimus dorsi, biceps, posterior GH capsule, posterior shoulder muscles
- Muscle weakness, inhibition-common by themselves or associated with pain generators (serratus anterior-weak, inhibited-develops early in scapular injury, lower trapezius-weak, altered activation, rotator cuff-impingement, weakness, imbalance, core weakness-seen in as many as 50% of cases of dyskinesis, loss of voluntary control-altered activation-seen early in patients with periscapular pain of any origin).

Frequently dyskinesis related to a pathoanatomical cause will have elements of pathophysiology that will need to be addressed in addition to restoring the anatomy.

PREVALENCE/INCIDENCE

The exact incidence of clinically significant scapular dyskinesis is not known. There are many reasons for this deficit, including different methods of definition and evaluation of dyskinesis, differences in targeted populations, and reliance on clinical methods of qualitative observational examination, which may lead to variable measurements. Most studies point to a high incidence of dyskinesis in populations that require repetitive overhead motions in their activities.[8] Sports including baseball, tennis, swimming, volleyball, cricket, kayaking, and surfing have shown an incidence of

30% to 70% dyskinesis.[9–15] Studies in symptomatic patients reveal an incidence between 64% and 100% depending on the anatomic diagnosis.[16]

PATIENT EVALUATION OVERVIEW

Because of the complexity of the possible scapular positions and motions in function and dysfunction, the scapula's role in the kinetic chain, and the multiple possible causative factors for dyskinesis, the clinical evaluation will need to be a step-wise, comprehensive process, using screening tests and maneuvers and employing more in-depth examination to evaluate the deficits identified by the screening tests. It should evaluate not only for the pathoanatomy, but also for the pathophysiology. It is a three-step process (**Fig. 1**). The first is the establishment of the presence or absence of dyskinesis, using the scapular dyskinesis test.[17,18] The second is establishing the relationship between the observed dyskinesis and the clinical symptoms using the corrective maneuvers, the Scapular Assistance Test (SAT) and the Scapular Retraction Test (SRT) and the Low Row maneuver.[5,7,19] The third is the evaluation of the possible causative factors, using standard testing.

Determination of the presence or absence of dyskinesis can be accomplished through observational evaluation of resting and dynamic scapular motion and position.[20] The patient's resting posture should be checked for side-to-side asymmetry and especially for evidence of a SICK position or inferomedial or medial border prominence. Clinical testing is performed by visual observation of static position at rest with arms at the side and dynamic arm motion using the Scapular Dyskinesis Test (SDT) (**Fig. 2**).[17,18] The exam is conducted by having the patients raise the arms in forward

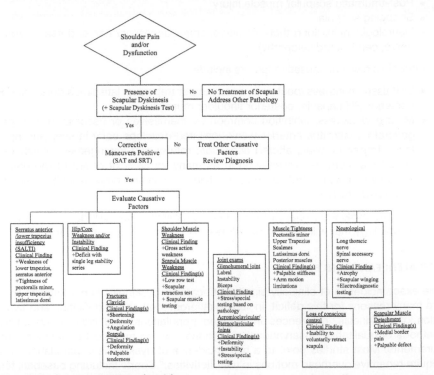

Fig. 1. Scapular examination algorithm.

flexion to maximum elevation, and then lower them three to five times. If the clinician is unsure the movement is altered or asymmetric, placing 3- to 5-pound weights in each hand can help accentuate possible alterations of motion.[17,18] Prominence of any aspect of the medial scapular border or inferior angle on the symptomatic side is recorded as "yes" (prominence detected) or "no" (prominence not detected).[20] The relationship of the dyskinesis to the clinical symptoms can be assessed through the scapular correctives maneuvers, the SAT, the SRT, and the Low Row Test.

In the SAT, the examiner applies gentle pressure to assist scapular upward rotation and posterior tilt as the patient elevates the arm (**Fig. 3**). A positive result occurs when the painful arc of impingement symptoms is relieved, and the arc of motion is increased. In the SRT, the examiner grades flexion strength using standard manual muscle testing procedures or evaluates labral injury in association with the modified dynamic labral shear test.[21] The examiner then places and manually stabilizes the scapula in a retracted position (**Fig. 4**). A positive test occurs when demonstrated flexion strength is increased or the symptoms of internal impingement related to possible labral injury are relieved in the retracted position. The Low Row Test can be used to assess the integrity of the lower trapezius and serratus anterior muscles.[22] To perform this maneuver, the patient is standing with the involved arm resting at the side with the palm facing posteriorly. The patient is instructed to extend their trunk and push their hand maximally against an examiner's resistance in the direction of shoulder extension and instructed to retract and depress the scapula (**Fig. 5**). This maneuver assesses both muscles' ability to actively stabilize the scapula while providing the examiner a visual depiction of lower trapezius muscle contraction. Although a positive SAT, SRT, or Low Row is not diagnostic for a specific form of shoulder pathology, it shows that scapular dyskinesis is involved in producing the symptoms, and that more detailed evaluations should be done to discover the causative factor(s) and indicates the need for early scapular rehabilitation exercises to improve scapular control.

The evaluation for the causative factors uses standard physical exam testing procedures. A general guide would include:

- Screening evaluation for hip/core stability and strength, using one leg stance and one leg squat evaluation
- Observation and palpation for medial scapula border tenderness and/or muscle defect
- Testing for periscapular and shoulder muscle voluntary activation and strength and ability to fully retract the scapula, using standard clinical tests
- Flexibility testing for commonly tight muscles including pectoralis minor, upper trapezius, and latissimus dorsi
- GH joint testing, including alteration of internal and external and horizontal adduction/abduction range of motion, anterior and posterior instability, labral injury, biceps injury, and rotator cuff disease, using standard exam techniques
- Clavicle, AC, and sternoclavicular joint evaluation for joint stability and bone shortening, angulation, or malrotation
- Neurological evaluation

The patient evaluation pathway can identify the pathoanatomical and pathophysiological factors underlying the observed alterations of position and motion. An unpublished study of 462 consecutive patients with shoulder pain who met the algorithm stage 1 and stage 2 criteria revealed that 35% of the patients had a pathoanatomical basis for their dyskinesis, whereas 65% had a pathophysiological basis. These findings suggest two-part outcomes result for patients with observed scapular dyskinesis that can be linked to the clinical symptoms. Treatment for those patients whose

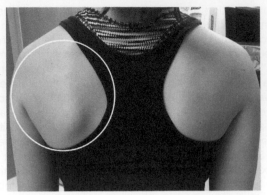

Fig. 2. Example of scapular dyskinesis with medial border and inferior angle prominence.

dyskinesis is secondary to identified pathoanatomy may include rehabilitation but frequently will require surgical means of restoration of the anatomy. Those whose dyskinesis is secondary to pathophysiology will need a comprehensive evaluation process to understand the muscular alterations that will serve as the basis for treatment.

SURGICAL TREATMENT

Many dyskinesis cases resulting from pathoanatomical causative factors may need restoration of the optimal anatomy to help create the proper mechanics. In addition, criteria for return to play or work should include the demonstration that normal scapular kinematics are present.

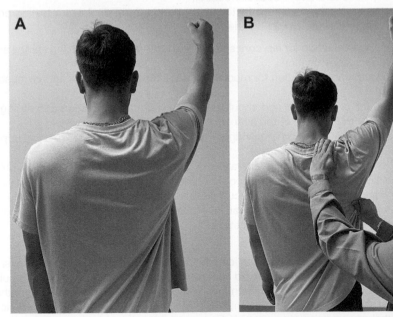

Fig. 3. Scapular Assistance Test (SAT)—The patient actively elevates the arm (*A*) then the scapula is stabilized with one hand and the other hand "assists" the scapula through its correct motion plane (*B*).

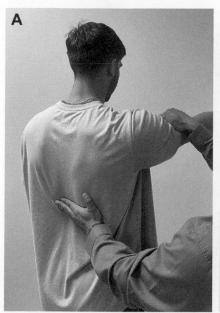 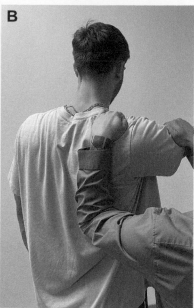

Fig. 4. Scapular Retraction Test (SRT)—The examiner first performs a traditional flexion manual strength test (*A*). The examiner stabilizes the medial border of the scapula and repeats the test; if the impingement symptoms are relieved and strength improved, the test is positive (*B*).

Neurologically Based

Surgery may be indicated for a patient with long thoracic nerve palsy after 1 year of symptoms and functional deficits, with no sign of recovery. Transfer of the sterno-costal head of the pectoralis major has been the most successful procedure, with generally favorable results.[23] The selected portion of the tendon is reflected from its insertion on the humerus, tunneled ventral to the scapula, and attached to the inferior angle of the scapula by one of several techniques. The tendon length generally requires augmentation with fascia lata or other graft for length. Surgery for spinal accessory nerve palsy surgery can be considered if nonsurgical management is unsuccessful. In the Eden-Lange transfer, which is intended to provide a dynamic medial and superior restraint, the levator scapula and rhomboids are transferred approximately 5 cm laterally and secured through drill holes to improve mechanical advantage and a substitute for trapezius function.[24] A recent modification of the Eden Lange transfer, which involves a more superior transfer of the rhomboids and more closely replicates the direction of pull of the lower trapezius, has been shown to have superior outcomes.[25]

Snapping Scapula

Snapping scapula is a descriptive term for painful crepitus along the medial scapular border during arm motion. Alterations in normal SHR underlie most incidences of snapping scapula.[26,27] but through creating increased compressive pressure along the medial border can produce pathoanatomy that contributes to the symptoms. Surgery may be indicated for a patient who has undergone a thorough but unsuccessful program of nonsurgical management. Good success rates have been reported with both open and arthroscopic techniques despite wide variance in techniques.[23,26]

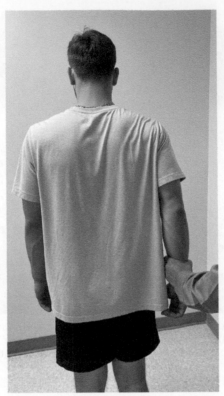

Fig. 5. In the Low Row Test, the arm is slightly extended and first tested without gluteal contraction then followed up with re-testing with gluteal contraction.

INTRA-ARTICULAR INJURIES AND ROTATOR CUFF INJURIES

Glenoid labral, biceps, and GH instability cases, and rotator cuff injuries, should be addressed by standard surgical techniques. The restoration of the anatomy may result in restoration of the normal kinematics, but more frequently rehabilitation will be required to restore the normal muscle activation patterns that will restore the kinematics. In nontraumatic GH injuries, especially labral injuries, the dyskinesis that has been found in association with a large percentage of the cases will need to be addressed so that the altered kinematics will not result in subsequent re-injury.

ACROMIOCLAVICULAR JOINT INSTABILITY AND CLAVICLE OR SCAPULAR FRACTURES

Surgical treatment should be designed to reconstruct and re-establish the strut function of the clavicle and the coupled AC ligamentous structures that stabilize joint function and control scapular motion. Multiple techniques have been advocated, but the procedure of choice should address and restore the clavicular shortening and/or malrotation and the ligament integrity that creates three-dimensional AC pathomechanics resulting from the injury that can affect scapular kinematics. Restoration of the scapular position and motion should be one of the outcomes of the treatment.[28]

Post-Traumatic Scapular Muscle Injury (Scapular Muscle Detachment)

Scapular muscle detachment is an uncommon but very painful and debilitating injury that results from a tensile load on the scapular supporting muscles, mainly involving the lower trapezius and the rhomboids. Early recognition of this injury can result in early treatment which can minimize the deleterious effects of the chronic pain on patient outcomes.[29,30] If patients have failed an appropriate scapular rehabilitation program, surgical reattachment is indicated. This is accomplished by direct reattachment through pairs of drill holes in the medial scapular border and scapular spine.[29,31] The detached and scarred rhomboids are mobilized and reattached onto the dorsal aspect of the scapula approximately 1 cm from the medial edge. The lower trapezius is mobilized and reattached along the proximal scapular spine.

NONSURGICAL TREATMENT
Is This Nerve Related?

Scapular dysfunction accompanied by moderate to severe pain with overt scapular dyskinesis and limited use of the arm can be due to multiple factors. The most typical factors are neurological damage (long thoracic or spinal accessory nerve palsies), traumatic injury (detachment of one or more scapular muscles), or chronic adaptations from unresolved injury, impairment, or soft tissue dysfunction. In cases of scapular dysfunction with neurologically rooted causes, rehabilitation can be performed to restore some level of arm function. Conservative treatment is recommended as most cases of long thoracic nerve injury are neuropraxic and will recover spontaneously. Because the nerve is so long, however, the recovery may be up to two years. It is for this reason that standardized protocols are difficult to develop and recommend. A general guideline would be (1) Verify neurological injury with electrodiagnostic testing; (2) If electrodiagnostic evidence exists that nerve injury is present, modify activity for 2 to 3 months to reduce movements that would tax or traction the affected nerve(s) and only consider immobilization if the patient has the potential to be noncompliant with activity restrictions; (3) Perform follow-up electrodiagnostic testing to determine if the nerve injury is improving (Recovery can be followed clinically, or via serial electromyography studies conducted no more frequently than every 3 months); and (4) Begin rehabilitation cautiously taking care not to use long lever arm movements in the early phases of treatment. Approximately 80% of patients do well in the long term with resolution of the winging and normal flexion and abduction, however many patients still have pain at long-term follow-up.[32] However, if the conservative measures fail, surgical options, such as muscle transfers may need to be considered.

Is This Soft Tissue Related?

Detecting musculoskeletal impairments requires clinicians to use multiple examination components and results to compile a clinical profile for the identification of scapular dyskinesis. Clinicians are recommended to follow the philosophy that the examination should guide the treatment.[33,34] For example, if altered scapular motion is identified via the SDT, the clinician should initially identify the specific observable components (ie, medial border prominence and scapular body positioning) and simultaneously consider what is the likely cause of the alteration (ie, deficiencies in mobility, strength, and/or motor control versus overt anatomical injury). The additional examination components of the corrective maneuvers, mobility testing, strength testing, and kinetic chain testing would help the clinician better identify the contributing cause. Once the cause is identified, the treatment plan can be optimized to target the cause(s). Let's consider the following case: A patient with shoulder pain has been noted to have scapular dyskinesis. The clinician observes the involved arm has a visible limitation of arm elevation (approximately 30° difference from the non-involved arm) and there is observed medial border and inferior angle prominence during the descent of the arm from the elevated position. The remainder of the examination reveals: palpable rigidity of the pectoralis minor, scapular movement during manual muscle testing of the serratus anterior and middle/lower trapezius both graded as 4/5, and negative special testing for all GH joint pathology. The combination of limited motion and a demonstrable strength decrease lead the clinician to suggest a treatment program focused on improving mobility and strength which based on the examination results would be an appropriate treatment pathway. However, the "how-to" of the treatment pathway should be considered.

Using this case as a guide, it would be common for interventions such as stretching, massage, and/or joint mobilization to be employed for addressing the mobility deficit while therapeutic exercises that have been shown to elicit high levels of muscle activity in specific muscles[35–37] to be used for addressing the strength deficit. However, various reports have noted that mobility and strength enhancement interventions have little influence on the scapular motion itself.[38–41] One point to consider is that mobility alterations are rarely acute in the scapula and/or shoulder. Although an acute decrease in GH rotation is common in overhead athletes following a throwing episode/exposure,[42–47] this phenomenon does not occur as often in the general population. Mobility deficits tend to manifest over time as it takes many weeks/months to create bony adaptations, capsular thickening, and various types of tendon responses to loading.[48] Although immediate gains in motion have been reported following the application of manual therapy interventions, the gains have not been shown to be long lasting.[49–57] The consensus within the literature is that these interventions positively impact pain and self-reported function which is more likely rooted in the neurophysiological effects related to endogenous pain control.[54] Thus, clinicians should educate patients that mobility interventions will likely be most effective when employed across multiple weeks and treatment sessions, and any immediate gains are likely not due to tissue correction/restoration.

When discussing therapeutic exercise selection, therapeutic exercises designed to target the specific shoulder and scapular muscles have been well described but these targeted exercises were primarily determined with electromyographic methodologies.[35–37,58–61] Although electromyography has helped identify which positions and maneuvers bias specific muscles, a common misconception from these results is that muscles can be isolated in rehabilitation. The complexities of shoulder/scapular architecture and movement do not allow any one muscle to be isolated during times of examination or treatment. Furthermore, various works have helped illustrate the summation of the activation phenomenon known as the kinetic chain which refutes the occurrence of isolated muscle activation.[62–70] Finally, the identified maneuvers were often performed in an isolated manner with the body in vertical or horizontal (prone or supine) stationary positions. These positions could lead to a less-than-optimal rehabilitation outcome likely due to the encouragement of inefficient or improper motor patterns.[7,71–75]

If mobility and strength are to be addressed during rehabilitation, there are additional guidelines to consider. A kinetic chain rehabilitation framework for shoulder dysfunction describes a rehabilitation approach that addresses mobility and strength but focuses on three critical characteristics.[76] First, patients perform exercises in upright positions rather than supine or prone positions to simulate functional demands. Second, the lever arm on the shoulder and trunk is shortened to reduce the load and torque on the injured arm. The exercises shown to elicit high amounts of muscle activity require the arm to be

Table 1
Nonoperative rehabilitation guidelines

Guideline	Key Points
Begin incorporating therapeutic exercise for addressing proximal segment control	Use exercises designed for leg and trunk/core strengthening Re-evaluate every few weeks to determine if strength is advancing
Employ exercises for scapular and shoulder mobility and/or lower extremity mobility as needed	Mobility can be addressed simultaneously with proximal segment control interventions Employ conscious correction (**Fig. 6**) with an appropriate type of feedback (visual, auditory, and/or kinesthetic)
Progress to short-lever interventions beginning with maneuvers that use trunk and leg motion to facilitate more optimal scapular positioning and mobility	These maneuvers will be performed sitting or standing and with the arm close to the trunk Examples: Low row (**Fig. 7**), Lawnmower with arm close to body (**Fig. 8**), Robbery (**Fig. 9**) Progress to the next guideline with visually observed improved scapular control and when patient can complete without early fatigue or symptom exacerbation
Phase out short-lever interventions and phase in long-lever maneuvers	Begin with maneuvers requiring the arm to be slightly flexed or abducted (approximately 30° to 45°) (**Figs. 10** and **11**) then transition to maneuvers with the arm at or above shoulder height (**Fig. 12**)

maintained in a set position throughout a range of motion and involve the arm to be further away from the body (also known as long lever exercises) thus increasing the demands on the muscles, that is, increased force output and torque generation.[61] Conversely, exercises that are performed with the elbow in 90° of flexion and/or with the arm close to the body (ie, short lever exercises) elicit lower levels of muscle activity and have decreased demands on the muscles.[22,77] Either long lever or short lever exercises are acceptable to use in rehabilitation however, the timing of implementation may cause different outcomes. Owing to the physical demands of long lever exercises, patients may experience irritation or soreness during or after the performance of the maneuvers when they are employed early in the rehabilitation process. In addition, it is also assumed that the greater demands require more effort be exerted to perform the exercises which may conflict with a patient attempting to establish scapular control. This could potentially create a situation where the patient becomes fatigued early in treatment sessions which in turn could cause the patient to use compensatory movement patterns during exercise performance. This would be counter-intuitive to the goal of establishing scapular control. Short lever exercises allow patients to focus on the stability function of the scapula and can often be performed with greater ease compared with long lever exercises. Finally, arm motions should be initiated using the legs and trunk to facilitate activation of the scapula and shoulder muscles, which is a typical motor pattern of motion. This framework has been previously described to include a set of progressive goals:[78] (1) establish proper postural alignment and motion; (2) facilitation of scapular motion via exaggeration of lower extremity/trunk movement; (3) exaggeration of scapular retraction in controlling excessive protraction; (4) use the closed chain exercise early; and (5) work in multiple planes.

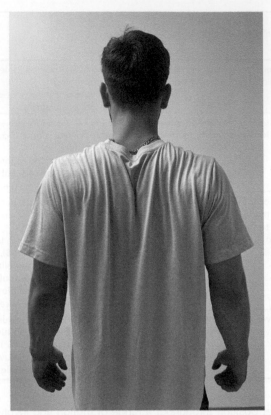

Fig. 6. Conscious correction of scapula begins with the patient standing and being instructed to actively "squeeze your shoulder blades together." Utilization of mirrors or mobile devices can assist patients with visualizing correct scapular positioning.

The complexity of scapular motion and the integrated relationship between the scapula, humerus, trunk, and legs suggest a need to develop rehabilitation programs that involve all segments working as a unit rather than isolated components. Obtaining mobility early in the rehabilitation would in turn allow for more fluid, task-specific movements to occur. Furthermore, integrating the legs and trunk more often in the rehabilitation process (as allowed by the patient's impairments and/or injury) would closely mimic activities of daily living, sports, and work tasks. The integrated approach expands the traditional focus of mobility and strength to also include enhancements in motor control thus improving rehabilitation outcomes.

TREATMENT RESISTANCE/COMPLICATIONS
Consider a Motor Control Approach

The aforementioned treatment approach that centers on mobility and strength improvement has been described based on the concept of scapular dyskinesis being the result of soft-tissue deficiencies.[7,22,38,39,41,76–87] However, various reports have noted that mobility and strength enhancement interventions have little influence on the scapular motion itself.[38–41] In addition to the concerns of chronicity of tissue alterations and the immediate false-positive effects of manual therapy on mobility as well

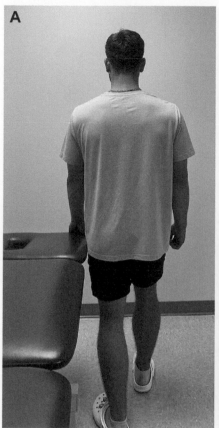
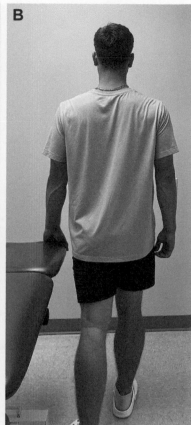

Fig. 7. For the low row, the patient is positioned standing with the hand of the involved arm against the side of a firm surface and legs slightly flexed (*A*). The patient should be instructed to extend the hips and trunk to facilitate scapular retraction and hold the contraction for 5 s (*B*).

as using muscle activity studies as the sole evidence for selecting exercises for rehabilitation, a recent clinical review suggested motor control has been lacking as a point of focus in scapular-based rehabilitation programs with the motor control principle of feedback being overlooked most often.[33]

The type and amount of feedback a person receives during task performance can positively influence the outcome of the task.[75,88–90] In most upper extremity tasks, visual feedback is used for joint positioning and error correction. However, because the posteriorly positioned scapula cannot be visualized, it is possible that the lack of visual feedback leads to the alterations in motion that manifests as scapular dyskinesis. Previous reports have shown intentional attempts at repositioning the scapula before elevating and/or rotating the humerus, called conscious correction/scapular squeezing/scapular setting, increases scapular muscle activity and enhances scapular kinematics.[71,73,75] Most clinicians have used "scapular squeezing" as an exercise but experience has shown that little instruction beyond "squeeze your shoulder blades together" is rarely conveyed to the patient. It is quite common for patients to "shrug" or simply be unable to perform this maneuver correctly, forcing clinicians to closely

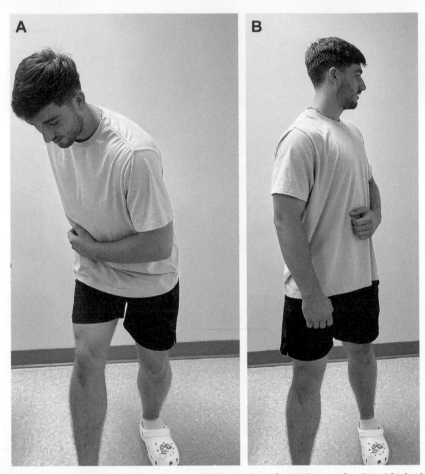

Fig. 8. Lawnmower with the arm close to body requires the patient to begin with the hips and trunk flexed and the arm held secure to the body (A). The patient is instructed to extend the hips and trunk, maintain the arm position next to the body, and followed by rotation of the trunk to facilitate scapular retraction (B).

monitor the motion for potential errant movements. It is possible that patients struggle with performing conscious scapular correction properly not only because of the scapula's posterior placement, but also because scapular motion is mostly characterized as accessory motion (ie, involuntary motion). Visual acuity is the strongest type of feedback humans use for knowledge of results, knowledge of performance, and overall motor control. Although non-adolescent patients can benefit from verbal external feedback provided by the clinician, there is a balance between too little and too much feedback that must be defined. Too little feedback does not inform the patient of occurring motion errors while too much feedback creates a dependency of the patient on the verbal feedback not allowing learning to occur.

In regard to scapular function, visual feedback,[91–95] auditory feedback,[91,92] and kinesthetic feedback[91,92] have been shown to positively influence scapular muscle activity and positioning. Considering the scapula as a "link" within the kinetic chain, the feedback approach may be better suited for re-establishing scapular control compared with the traditional mobility and strength focus as feedback relates to the

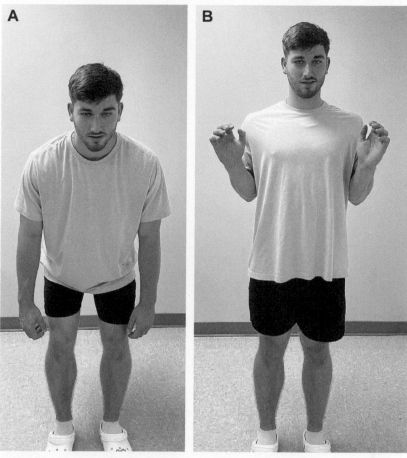

Fig. 9. Robbery maneuver begins with the knees and trunk slightly flexed (*A*) and is performed by instructing the patient to "place the elbows in the back pockets" (*B*).

sequential activation within the kinetic chain. Combining the kinetic chain approach described earlier with feedback serves as an integrated approach where the patient is required to perform exercises from a sitting or standing position to perform (and learn) the necessary motor patterns that require integrated use of the majority of the kinetic chain segments (ie, using the legs and trunk to facilitate scapular and shoulder movement and muscle activation).[22,77,96–99] However, there are no empirical reports or randomized control trials that have compared a motor control/kinetic chain focused program against a program that does not use this approach. To date, general guidelines for program development have been suggested including[33]:

- Short lever progression beginning with the arm close to the body and then progressively advancing the arm to angles further away from the body
- Sitting and standing preferred over prone or supine exercises
- Target impairments in the order of mobility, motor control, strength, and endurance but allow the examination to guide the treatment
- Use longer lever maneuvers later in the rehabilitation program
- Advance to plyometric-based maneuvers just before discharge

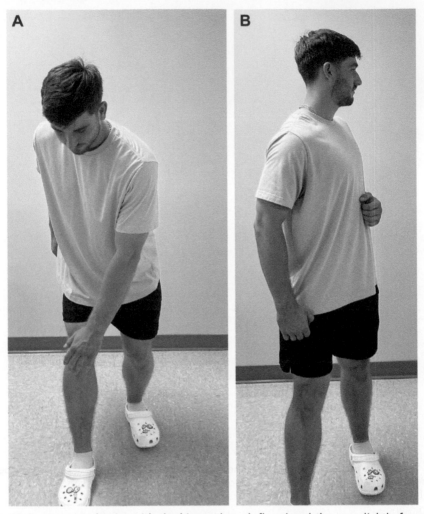

Fig. 10. Lawnmower begins with the hips and trunk flexed and the arm slightly forward elevated (*A*). The patient is instructed to extend the hips and trunk, followed by rotation of the trunk to facilitate scapular retraction (*B*).

A sample program has been provided in **Table 1**. Dosage recommendations include beginning with 1 to 2 sets of 5 to 10 repetitions with no external resistance. Additional sets and repetitions can be added based on symptoms and exercise tolerance, with a goal of 5 to 6 sets of 10 repetitions being able to be performed without an increase in symptoms before adding resistance. Resistance may be added next beginning with light free weights (2 to 3 pounds maximum) and then progressing to elastic resistance. The stability of free weights allows those devices to be used before elastic resistance because elastic resistance, although effective at increasing scapular muscle activity,[98] has high variability when used by patients, especially when arm position is progressed throughout a treatment program.[100] If elastic resistance were to be used, it can be adequately monitored and progressed using perceived exertion scales.[101] Feedback may be incorporated throughout the treatment program but there is not an exclusive

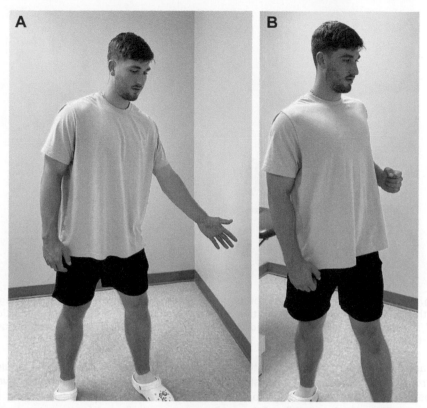

Fig. 11. Fencing maneuver begins in a standing position with the patient grasping resistance bands or tubing (*A*). It uses multiple kinetic chain segments to enhance proper muscle scapular muscle activation through activation of the legs, trunk, scapula, and arm (*B*).

type to recommend considering various forms of feedback have been shown to have positive clinical influence.[91–95] However, it should be noted that too much feedback can be detrimental to learning as the patient becomes reliant on the knowledge of performance.[88]

NEW DEVELOPMENTS

Although clinicians can become well trained at distinguishing between clinically significant and benign scapular dyskinesis,[17,18] the inherent flaw with observational analysis is the natural subjectivity of the assessment method. Multiple methods of quantitative analysis have been proposed but have not been found to be clinically useful due to lack of consistent reliability,[102,103] limitation of data to one scapular kinematic component,[104–107] large error of the data in relation to actual bone motion,[108–110] or inability to use the assessment method(s) in a clinical setting due to inconveniences of cost and set-up (bone pins, electromagnetic tracking, computed tomography scans).[111–114] As a result, even with the known limitations,[115,116] the visual observational method is still the most frequently selected by clinicians to identify the presence or absence of dyskinesis in the evaluation of the patient,[117] and to make generalized assessments of change during the treatment process. Precise and effective quantitative assessment of scapular motion in the clinical setting that encompasses all

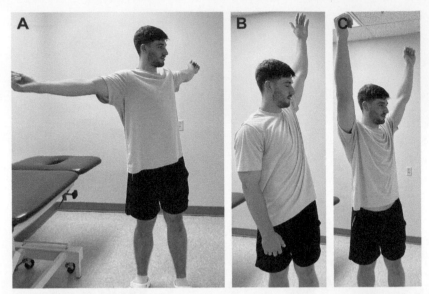

Fig. 12. T's, I's, and Y's with trunk rotation are standing rotator cuff exercises that begin with the patient in an upright position with the arms transitioning through abduction (*A*), forward elevation (*B*), and elevation in the plane of the scapula (*C*) while simultaneously performing trunk rotation.

scapular kinematic components of three-dimensional motion by a device that contains gyroscopic technology and/or a system of wearable sensors are currently being developed[118–123]; however, although psychometrics have been reported as being at acceptable levels, the novelty of the systems have not allowed for rigorous clinical testing to provide clinically useful recommendations at this time.

SUMMARY/DISCUSSION/FUTURE DIRECTIONS

Scapular dyskinesis is an impairment that has causative factors, and those factors should be discerned from a comprehensive physical examination. The examination should not exclude assessments related to identifying pathoanatomical causes but the pathoanatomical approach should not be the primary focus of the examination. Using clinician experience and the best available evidence, a qualitative examination for determining the presence or absence of a scapular contribution to shoulder dysfunction is currently the best option widely available to clinicians. Future investigations should attempt to standardize methodological approaches to perform better comparisons between studies and generate higher quality results. Finally, rehabilitation approaches should be reconsidered where enhancing motor control becomes the primary focus rather than primarily increasing mobility and strength.

CLINICS CARE POINTS

- Make the comprehensive diagnosis-rule in or rule out scapular dyskinesis in patients with shoulder or arm pain.
- Use the clinical pathway to develop the information needed to initiate the first treatment steps.

- Only one-third of the patients with demonstrated dyskinesis have a pathoanatomical cause for the dyskinesis. Pathophysiological causes, which can also create the altered kinematics need to be evaluated as well.

- Understand that demonstrated peri scapular muscle weakness may be secondary to inhibition rather than strictly a strength deficit.

- The complexity of scapular motion and the integrated relationship between the scapula, humerus, trunk, and legs suggest a need to develop rehabilitation programs that involve all segments working as a unit rather than isolated components.

- Addressing deficits in mobility and strength may be necessary but including motor control enhancement should also be considered.

DISCLOSURE

W. Ben Kibler, J.W. Lockhart, and A. Sciascia are paid consultants for Alyve Medical, Inc. W. Ben Kibler and Aaron Sciascia receive royalties from Springer Publishing for coediting two textbooks.

REFERENCES

1. Veeger HEJ, van der Helm FCT. Shoulder function: the perfect compromise between mobility and stability. J Biomech 2007;40:2119–29.
2. Dvir Z, Berme N. The shoulder complex in elevation of the arm: a mechanism approach. J Biomech 1978;11:219–25.
3. Kibler WB, Sciascia AD. Current concepts: scapular dyskinesis. Br J Sports Med 2010;44(5):300–5.
4. Burkhart SS, Morgan CD, Kibler WB. The disabled throwing shoulder: spectrum of pathology Part III: The SICK scapula, scapular dyskinesis, the kinetic chain, and rehabilitation. Arthroscopy 2003;19(6):641–61.
5. Kibler WB, Ludewig PM, McClure PW, et al. Scapula summit 2009. J Orthop Sports Phys Ther 2009;39(11):A1–13.
6. Moore-Reed SD, Kibler WB, Sciascia AD, et al. Preliminary development of a clinical prediction rule for treatment of patients with suspected SLAP tears. Arthroscopy 2014;30(12):1540–9.
7. Kibler WB, Ludewig PM, McClure PW, et al. Clinical implications of scapular dyskinesis in shoulder injury: The 2013 consensus statement from the "scapula summit". Br J Sports Med 2013;47:877–85.
8. Burn MB, McCulloch PC, Lintner DM, et al. Prevalence of scapular dyskinesis in overhead and nonoverhead athletes. Orthop J Sports Med 2016;4. 2325967115627608.
9. Gomes BN, Schell MS, Gomes Rosa C, et al. Prevalence of scapular dyskinesis and shoulder pain in amateur surfers from Rio Grande do Sul: a cross-sectional study. Fisioter Pesqui 2020;27:293–8.
10. Johannsson A, Svantesson U, Tannerstedt J, et al. Prevalence of shoulder pain in Swedish flatwater kayakers and its relation to range of motion and scapula stability of the shoulder joint. J Sports Sci 2016;34:951–8.
11. Laxmi R, Prosenjit P, Shahid MD. Prevalence of shoulder injuries and altered scapular positioning in young elite cricketers. Int J Sport Sci Fit 2015;5:130–61.
12. Madsen PH, Bak K, Jensen S, et al. Training induces scapular dyskinesis in pain-free competitive swimmers: a reliability and observational study. Clin J Sport Med 2011;21(2):109–13.

13. Maor MB, Ronin T, Kalichman L. Scapular dyskinesis among competitive swimmers. J Bodywork Move Ther 2017;21:633–6.
14. Reeser JC, Joy EA, Porucznik CA, et al. Risk factors for volleyball-related shoulder pain and dysfunction. Phys Med Rehabil 2010;2(1):27–35.
15. Silva RT, Hartmann LG, Laurino CF, et al. Clinical and ultrasonographic correlation between scapular dyskinesia and subacromial space measurement among junior elite tennis players. Br J Sports Med 2010;44(6):407–10.
16. Warner JJP, Micheli LJ, Arslanian LE, et al. Scapulothoracic motion in normal shoulders and shoulders with glenohumeral instability and impingement syndrome. Clin Orthop Rel Res 1992;285(191):199.
17. McClure PW, Tate AR, Kareha S, et al. A clinical method for identifying scapular dyskinesis: part 1: reliability. J Athl Train 2009;44(2):160–4.
18. Tate AR, McClure PW, Kareha S, et al. A clinical method for identifying scapular dyskinesis: part 2: validity. J Athl Train 2009;44(2):165–73.
19. Kibler WB. The role of the scapula in athletic function. Am J Sports Med 1998; 26:325–37.
20. Uhl TL, Kibler WB, Gecewich B, et al. Evaluation of clinical assessment methods for scapular dyskinesis. Arthroscopy 2009;25(11):1240–8.
21. Kibler WB, Sciascia AD, Dome DC. Evaluation of apparent and absolute supraspinatus strength in patients with shoulder injury using the scapular retraction test. Am J Sports Med 2006;34(10):1643–7.
22. Kibler WB, Sciascia AD, Uhl TL, et al. Electromyographic analysis of specific exercises for scapular control in early phases of shoulder rehabilitation. Am J Sports Med 2008;36(9):1789–98.
23. Steinman S, Wood M. Pectoralis major transfer for serratus anterior paralysis. J Shoulder Elbow Surg 2003;12:555–60.
24. Romero J, Gerber C. Levator scapulae and rhomboid transfer for paralysis of trapezius: the Eden-Lange procedure. J Bone Joint Surg Br 2003;85(8):1141–5.
25. Elhassan BT, Wagner ER. Outcome of triple-tendon transfer, an Eden-Lange variant, to reconstruct trapezius paralysis. J Shoulder Elbow Surg 2015;24: 1307–13.
26. Kuhne M, Boniquit N, Ghodadra N, et al. The snapping scapula: diagnosis and treatment. Arthroscopy 2009;25(11):1298–311.
27. Gaskill T, Millett PJ. Snapping scapula syndrome: diagnosis and management. J Am Acad Orthop Surg 2013;21(4):214–24.
28. Kibler WB, Sciascia AD, Morris BJ, et al. Treatment of symptomatic acromioclavicular joint instability by a docking technique: clinical indications, surgical technique, and outcomes. Arthroscopy 2017;33:696–708.
29. Kibler WB, Sciascia A, Uhl T. Medial scapular muscle detachment: clinical presentation and surgical treatment. J Shoulder Elbow Surg 2014;23(1):58–67.
30. Kibler WB, Jacobs CA, Sciascia AD. Pain catastrophizing behaviors and their relation to poor patient-reported outcomes after scapular muscle reattachment. J Shoulder Elbow Surg 2018;27:1564–71.
31. Kibler WB. Scapular surgery I-IV. In: Reider B, Terry MA, Provencher MT, editors. Sports medicine surgery. Philadelphia: Elsevier Saunders; 2010. p. 237–67, 978-1-4160-3277-9.
32. Pikkarainen V, Kettunen J, Vastamaki M. The natural course of serratus palsy at 2 to 31 years. Clin Orthop Rel Res 2013;471:1555–63.
33. Sciascia A, Kibler WB. Current views of scapular dyskinesis and its possible clinical relevance. Int J Sports Phys Ther 2022;17:117–30.

34. Ludewig PM, Kamonseki DH, Staker JL, et al. Changing our diagnostic paradigm: movement system diagnostic classification. Int J Sports Phys Ther 2017;12:884–93.
35. Blackburn TA, McLeod WD, White B, et al. EMG analysis of posterior rotator cuff exercises. Ath Train. Spring 1990;25(1):42–5, 40.
36. Townsend H, Jobe FW, Pink M, et al. Electromyographic analysis of the glenohumeral muscles during a baseball rehabilitation program. Am J Sports Med 1991;19:264–72.
37. Reinold MM, Wilk KE, Fleisig GS, et al. Electromyographic analysis of the rotator cuff and deltoid musculature during common shoulder external rotation exercises. J Orthop Sports Phys Ther 2004;34:385–94.
38. Haik MN, Alburquerque-Sendín F, Silva CZ, et al. Scapular kinematics pre- and post-thoracic thrust manipulation in individuals with and without shoulder impingement symptoms: a randomized controlled study. J Orthop Sports Phys Ther 2014;44:475–87.
39. Camargo PR, Alburquerque-Sendín F, Avila MA, et al. Effects of stretching and strengthening exercises, with and without manual therapy, on scapular kinematics, function, and pain in individuals with shoulder impingement: a randomized controlled trial. J Orthop Sports Phys Ther 2015;45:984–97.
40. Kardouni JR, Pidcoe PE, Shaffer SW, et al. Thoracic spine manipulation in individuals with subacromial impingement syndrome does not immediately alter thoracic spine kinematics, thoracic excursion, or scapular kinematics: a randomized controlled trial. J Orthop Sports Phys Ther 2015;45:527–38.
41. Rosa DP, Borstad JD, Pogetti LS, et al. Effects of a stretching protocol for the pectoralis minor on muscle length, function, and scapular kinematics in individuals with and without shoulder pain. J Hand Ther 2017;30:20–9.
42. Reinold MM, Wilk KE, Macrina LC, et al. Changes in shoulder and elbow passive range of motion after pitching in professional baseball players. Am J Sports Med 2008;36(3):523–7.
43. Kibler WB, Sciascia AD, Moore SD. An acute throwing episode decreases shoulder internal rotation. Clin Orthop Rel Res 2012;470:1545–51.
44. Proske U, Morgan DL, Gregory JE. Thixotropy in skeletal muscle and in muscle spindles: a review. Progr Neurobiol 1993;41:705–21.
45. Proske U, Morgan DL. Do cross-bridges contribute to the tension during stretch of passive muscle? J Muscle Res Cell Motil 1999;20:433–42.
46. Proske U, Morgan DL. Muscle damage from eccentric exercise: mechanism, mechanical signs, adaptation and clinical applications. J Physiol 2001;537(2): 333–45.
47. Reisman S, Walsh LD, Proske U. Warm up stretches reduce sensations of stiffness and soreness after eccentric exercise. Med Sci Sport Exerc 2005;37: 929–36.
48. Manske R, Wilk KE, Davies G, et al. Glenohumeral motion deficits: friend or foe? Int J Sports Phys Ther 2013;8:537–53.
49. Manske RC, Meschke M, Porter A, et al. A randomized controlled single-blinded comparison of stretching versus stretching and joint mobilization for posterior shoulder tightness measured by internal rotation motion loss. Sports Health 2010;2(2):94–100.
50. Brudvig TJ, Kulkarni H, Shah S. The effect of therapeutic exercise and mobilization on patients with shoulder dysfunction: a systematic review with meta-analysis. J Orthop Sports Phys Ther 2011;41(10):734–48.

51. Harshbarger ND, Eppelheimer BL, Valovich McLeod TC, et al. The effectiveness of shoulder stretching and joint mobilizations on posterior shoulder tightness. J Sport Rehabil 2013;22(4):313–9.

52. Moon GD, Lim JY, Kim DY, et al. Comparison of Maitland and Kaltenborn mobilization techniques for improving shoulder pain and range of motion in frozen shoulders. J Phys Ther Sci 2015;27:1391–5.

53. Ho CYC, Sole G, Munn J. The effectiveness of manual therapy in the management of musculoskeletal disorders of the shoulder: a systematic review. Man Ther 2009;14:463–74.

54. Bialosky JE, Bishop MD, Price DD, et al. The mechanisms of manual therapy in the treatment of musculoskeletal pain: a comprehensive model. Man Ther 2009; 14:531–8.

55. Bronfort G, Haas M, Evans R, et al. Effectiveness of manual therapies: the UK evidence report. Chiro Osteo 2010;18:3.

56. Gebremariam L, Hay EM, van der Sande R, et al. Subacromial impingement syndrome—effectiveness of physiotherapy and manual therapy. Br J Sports Med 2014;48:1202–8.

57. Desjardins-Charbonneau A, Roy JS, Dionne CE, et al. The efficacy of manual therapy for rotator cuff tendinopathy: a systematic review and meta-analysis. J Orthop Sports Phys Ther 2015;45:330–50.

58. Moseley JB, Jobe FW, Pink MM, et al. EMG analysis of the scapular muscles during a shoulder rehabilitation program. Am J Sports Med 1992;20(2):128–34.

59. Hintermeister RA, Lange GW, Schultheis JM, et al. Electromyographic activity and applied load during shoulder rehabilitation exercises using elastic resistance. Am J Sports Med 1998;26(2):210–20.

60. Decker MJ, Hintermeister RA, Faber KJ, et al. Serratus anterior muscle activity during selected rehabilitation exercises. Am J Sports Med 1999;27(6):784–91.

61. Reinold MM, Escamilla R, Wilk KE. Current concepts in the scientific and clinical rationale behind exercises for glenohumeral and scapulothoracic musculature. J Orthop Sports Phys Ther 2009;39:105–17.

62. Toyoshima S, Hoshikawa T, Miyashita M. Contributions of body parts to throwing performance. In: Nelson RC, Morehouse CA, editors. Biomechanics IV. Baltimore: University Park Press; 1974. p. 169–74.

63. Hirashima M, Kadota H, Sakurai S, et al. Sequential muscle activity and its functional role in the upper extremity and trunk during overarm throwing. J Sport Sci 2002;20:301–10.

64. Hirashima M, Kudo K, Watarai K, et al. Control of 3D limb dynamics in unconstrained overarm throws of different speeds performed by skilled baseball players. J Neurophysiol 2007;97(1):680–91.

65. Hirashima M, Yamane K, Nakamura Y, et al. Kinetic chain of overarm throwing in terms of joint rotations revealed by induced acceleration analysis. J Biomech 2008;41:2874–83.

66. Putnam CA. Sequential motions of body segments in striking and throwing skills: description and explanations. J Biomech 1993;26:125–35.

67. Davids K, Glazier PS, Araujo D, et al. Movement systems as dynamical systems: the functional role of variability and its implications for sports medicine. Sports Med 2003;33(4):245–60.

68. Glazier PS, Davids K. Constraints on the complete optimization of human motion. Sports Med 2009;39(1):16–28.

69. Bouisset S, Zattara M. A sequence of postural movements precedes voluntary movement. Neurosci Let 1981;22:263–70.

70. Zattara M, Bouisset S. Posturo-kinetic organisation during the early phase of voluntary upper limb movement. 1 Normal subjects. J Neurol Neurosurg Psychiatr 1988;51:956–65.
71. De May K, Danneels L, Cagnie B, et al. Conscious correction of scapular orientation in overhead athletes performing selected shoulder rehabilitation exercises: the effect on trapezius muscle activation measured by surface electromyography. J Orthop Sports Phys Ther 2013;43(1):3–10.
72. Willmore EG, Smith MJ. Scapular dyskinesia: evolution towards a systems-based approach. Shoulder Elbow 2016;8:61–70.
73. Ou HL, Huang TS, Chen YT, et al. Alterations of scapular kinematics and associated muscle activation specific to symptomatic dyskinesis type after conscious control. Man Ther 2016;26:97–103.
74. Pires ED, Camargo PR. Analysis of the kinetic chain in asymptomatic individuals with and without scapular dyskinesis. Clin Biomech 2018;54:8–15.
75. Huang TS, Du WY, Wang TG, et al. Progressive conscious control of scapular orientation with video feedback has improvement in muscle balance ratio in patients with scapular dyskinesis: a randomized controlled trial. J Shoulder Elbow Surg 2018;27:1407–14.
76. McMullen J, Uhl TL. A kinetic chain approach for shoulder rehabilitation. J Ath Train 2000;35(3):329–37.
77. De May K, Daneels L, Cagnie B, et al. Kinetic chain influences on upper and lower trapezius muscle activation during eight variations of a scapular retraction exercise in overhead athletes. J Sci Med Sport 2013;16:65–70.
78. Sciascia A, Cromwell R. Kinetic chain rehabilitation: a theoretical framework. Rehabil Res Pract 2012;2012:1–9.
79. Sciascia AD, Thigpen CA, Namdari S, et al. Kinetic chain abnormalities in the athletic shoulder. Sports Med Arthrosc Rev 2012;20(1):16–21.
80. Kibler WB, Sciascia A, Wilkes T. Scapular dyskinesis and its relation to shoulder injury. J Am Acad Orthop Surg 2012;20(6):364–72.
81. Michener LA, Walsworth MK, Burnet EN. Effectiveness of rehabilitation for patients with subacromial impingement syndrome. J Hand Ther 2004;17:152–64.
82. Tate AR, McClure PW, Young IA, et al. Comprehensive impairment-based exercise and manual therapy intervention for patients with subacromial impingement syndrome: a case series. J Orthop Sports Phys Ther 2010;40(8):474–93.
83. Ellenbecker TS, Cools A. Rehabilitation of shoulder impingement syndrome and rotator cuff injuries: an evidence-based review. Br J Sports Med 2010;44:319–27.
84. Cools A, Johansson FR, Cagnie B, et al. Stretching the posterior shoulder structures in subjects with internal rotation deficit: Comparison of two stretching techniques. Shoulder and Elbow 2012;4(1):56–63.
85. De May K, Danneels L, Cagnie B, et al. Scapular muscle rehabilitation exercises in overhead athletes with impingement symptoms: effect of a 6-week training program on muscle recruitment and functional outcome. Am J Sports Med 2012;40(8):1906–15.
86. Borstad JD, Ludewig PM. The effect of long versus short pectoralis minor resting length on scapular kinematics in healthy individuals. J Orthop Sports Phys Ther 2005;35(4):227–38.
87. Borstad JD, Ludewig PM. Comparison of three stretches for the pectoralis minor muscle. J Shoulder Elbow Surg 2006;15(3):324–30.
88. Sanchez FJN, Gonzalez JG. Influence of three accuracy levels of knowledge of results on motor skill acquisition. J Hum Sport Exerc 2010;5(3):476–84.

89. Sidaway B, Bates J, Occhiogrosso B, et al. Interaction of feedback frequency and task difficulty in children's motor skill learning. Phys Ther 2012;92:948–57.

90. Ramachandran VS, Altschuler EL. The use of visual feedback, in particular mirror visual feedback, in restoring brain function. Brain 2009;132:1693–710.

91. Mottram SL, Woledge RC, Morrissey D. Motion analysis study of a scapular orientation exercise and subjects' ability to learn the exercise. Man Ther 2009; 14:13–8.

92. Worsley P, Warner M, Mottram S, et al. Motor control retraining exercises for shoulder impingement: effects on function, muscle activation, and biomechanics in young adults. J Shoulder Elbow Surg 2013;22:e11-e19.

93. Du WY, Huang TS, Chiu YC, et al. Single-session video and electromyography feedback in overhead athletes with scapular dyskinesis and impingement syndrome. J Ath Train 2020;55:265–73.

94. Antunes A, Carnide F, Matias R. Real-time kinematic biofeedback improves scapulothoracic control and performance during scapular-focused exercises: a single-blind randomized controlled laboratory study. Hum Mov Sci 2016;48: 44–53.

95. Weon JH, Kwon OY, Cynn HS, et al. Real-time visual feedback can be used to activate scapular upward rotators in people with scapular winging: an experimental study. J Physiother 2011;57:101–7.

96. Oliver GD, Plummer HA, Gascon SS. Electromyographic analysis of traditional and kinetic chain exercises for dynamic shoulder movements. J Strength Cond Res 2016;30:3146–54.

97. Oliver GD, Washington JK, Barfield JW, et al. Quantitative analysis of proximal and distal kinetic chain musculature during dynamic exercises. J Strength Cond Res 2018;32:1545–53.

98. Wasserberger KW, Downs JL, Barfield JW, et al. Lumbopelvic-hip complex and scapular stabilizing muscle activations during fullbody exercises with and without resistance bands. J Strength Cond Res 2020;34:2840–8.

99. De May K, Danneels L, Cagnie B, et al. Are kinetic chain rowing exercises relevant in shoulder and trunk injury prevention training? Br J Sports Med 2011; 45(4):320.

100. Tsuruike M, Ellenbecker TS, Kagaya Y, et al. Analysis of scapular muscle EMG activity during elastic resistance oscillation exercises from the perspective of different arm positions. Sports Health 2020;12:395–400.

101. Colado JC, Garcia-Masso X, Triplett TN, et al. Concurrent validation of the omniresistance exercise scale of perceived exertion with thera-band resistance bands. J Strength Cond Res 2012;26:3018–24.

102. Odom CJ, Hurd CE, Denegar CR, et al. Intratester and intertester reliability of the lateral scapular slide test and its ability to predict shoulder pathology. J Ath Train 1995;30(2):s9.

103. Odom CJ, Taylor AB, Hurd CE, et al. Measurement of scapular assymetry and assessment of shoulder dysfunction using the lateral scapular slide test: A reliability and validity study. Phys Ther 2001;81:799–809.

104. Scibek JS, Carcia CR. Assessment of scapulohumeral rhythm for scapular plane shoulder elevation using a modified digital inclinometer. World J Orthop 2012;3:87–94.

105. Scibek JS, Carcia CR. Validation of a new method for assessing scapular anterior-posterior tilt. Int J Sports Phys Ther 2014;9:644–56.

106. Watson L, Balster SM, Finch C, et al. Measurement of scapula upward rotation: a reliable clinical procedure. Br J Sports Med 2005;39:599–603.

107. Johnson MP, McClure PW, Karduna AR. New method to assess scapular upward rotation in subjects with shoulder pathology. J Orthop Sports Phys Ther 2001;31:81–9.
108. Johnson GR, Stuart PR. A method for the measurement of three-dimensional scapular movement. Clin Biomech 1993;8. 296-273.
109. van-der-Helm FC, Pronk GM. Three-dimensional recording and description of motions of the shoulder mechanism. J Biomech Eng 1995;117(1):27–40.
110. Lempereur M, Brochard S, Leboeuf F, et al. Validity and reliability of 3D marker based scapular motion analysis: a systematic review. J Biomech 2014;47(10): 2219–30.
111. McClure PW, Michener LA, Sennett BJ, et al. Direct 3-dimensional measurement of scapular kinematics during dynamic movements in vivo. J Shoulder Elbow Surg 2001;10:269–77.
112. Lawrence RL, Braman JP, LaPrade RF, et al. Comparison of 3-Dimensional shoulder complex kinematics in individuals with and without shoulder pain, part 1: sternoclavicular, acromioclavicular, and scapulothoracic joints. J Orthop Sports Phys Ther 2014;44:636–45.
113. Lawrence RL, Braman JP, Staker JL, et al. Comparison of 3-dimensional shoulder complex kinematics in individuals with and without shoulder pain, part 2: glenohumeral joint. J Orthop Sports Phys Ther 2014;44:646–55.
114. Ludewig PM, Phadke V, Braman JP, et al. Motion of the shoulder complex during multiplanar humeral elevation. J Bone Joint Surg Am 2009;91A(2):378–89.
115. D'hondt NE, Kiers H, Pool JJM, et al. Reliability of performance-based clinical measurements to assess shoulder girdle kinematics and positioning: systematic review. Phys Ther 2017;97:124–44.
116. D'hondt NE, Pool JJM, Kiers H, et al. Validity of clinical measurement instruments assessing scapular function: insufficient evidence to recommend any instrument for assessing scapular posture, movement, and dysfunction—a systematic review. J Orthop Sports Phys Ther 2020;50:632–41.
117. Larsen CM, Juul-Kristensen B, Lund H, et al. Measurement properties of existing clinical assessment methods evaluating scapular positioning and function. A systematic review. Physiother Theor Pract 2014;30:453–82.
118. Parel I, Cutti AG, Fiumana G, et al. Ambulatory measurement of the scapulo-humeral rhythm: Intra- and inter-operator agreement of a protocol based on inertial and magnetic sensors. Gait Posture 2012;35:636–40.
119. Pellegrini A, Tonino P, Paladini P, et al. Motion analysis assessment of alterations in the scapulo-humeral rhythm after throwing in baseball pitchers. Musculoskelet Surg 2013;97:S9–13.
120. Cutti AG, Parel I, Raggi M, et al. Prediction bands and intervals for the scapulo-humeral coordination based on the Bootstrap and two Gaussian methods. J Biomech 2014;47:1035–44.
121. Parel I, Cutti AG, Kraszewski A, et al. Intra-protocol repeatability and inter-protocol agreement for the analysis of scapulo-humeral coordination. Med Biol Eng Comput 2014;52:271–82.
122. Cutti AG, Parel I, Pellegrini A, et al. The Constant score and the assessment of scapula dyskinesis: Proposal and assessment of an integrated outcome measure. J Electromyogr Kinesiol 2016;29:81–9.
123. Silverson OA, Lemaster NG, Hettrich CM, et al. Reliability and validity of a clinical assessment tool for measuring scapular motion in all 3 anatomical planes. J Ath Train 2021;56:586–93.

Adhesive Capsulitis

Nels Leafblad, MD[a],*, Josh Mizels, MD[b], Robert Tashjian, MD[c],
Peter Chalmers, MD[c]

KEYWORDS

- Adhesive capsulitis • Arthroscopic capsular release • Range of motion
- Diabetes mellitus

KEY POINTS

- Risk factors for adhesive capsulitis (AC) include diabetes, thyroid disease, recent surgery, and perhaps COVID-19 infection.
- Limited shoulder active and passive range of motion (ROM), particularly external rotation and forward elevation, should raise suspicion for AC.
- Treatment with non-steroidal anti-inflammatory drug (NSAIDs), corticosteroid injection, and physical therapy should be implemented early in the disease process and this may shorten duration of symptoms.
- When nonoperative treatment fails, arthroscopic capsular release is a highly successful treatment option.

INTRODUCTION/BACKGROUND/PREVALENCE

Adhesive capsulitis (AC), colloquially known as "frozen shoulder," is a relatively common disorder, affecting approximately 2% to 5% of the general population.[1,2] The incidence may be higher as the condition can be relatively mild and self-limited, and thus, many patients who experience it may never present for treatment. It involves a pathologic process of gradual fibrosis of the glenohumeral (GH) joint that leads to limited active and passive range of motion (ROM), contracture of the joint capsule, and shoulder pain.[3] The condition was first described by Simon-Emmanuel Duplay, who named it "scapulohumeral periarthritis." It was Earnest Codman who later coined the term "frozen shoulder" in 1934, emphasizing the disabling loss of shoulder motion associated with the condition.[4] Julius Neviaser later redefined the condition as AC in 1945, as his histologic study elucidated the inflammatory and fibrotic changes observed in the capsule and adjacent bursa.[5,6]

a Department of Sports Medicine, University of Utah, 590 Wakara Way, Salt Lake City, UT 84108, USA; b Department of Orthopaedic Surgery, University of Utah, 590 Wakara Way, Salt Lake City, UT 84108, USA; c Department of Shoulder and Elbow Surgery, University of Utah, 590 Wakara Way, Salt Lake City, UT 84108, USA
* Corresponding author. 590 Wakara Way, Salt Lake City, UT 84108.
E-mail address: nels.leafblad@hsc.utah.edu

Phys Med Rehabil Clin N Am 34 (2023) 453–468
https://doi.org/10.1016/j.pmr.2022.12.009
1047-9651/23/© 2022 Elsevier Inc. All rights reserved.

AC is one of several stiff shoulder conditions and is typically thought of as an idiopathic condition. The stiff shoulder category also includes conditions such as postoperative stiffness, post-traumatic stiffness, and neurologic stiffness, which tend to have different treatments and prognoses than does AC. AC is generally regarded as a self-limiting process that resolves within 1 to 3 years, but symptoms have been known to last longer in 20% to 50% of patients.[7-9] There are nonoperative treatment options that may shorten the course of disease, and in patients with AC refractory to nonoperative management, open arthroscopic release is a safe and effective treatment option.

PATIENT EVALUATION OVERVIEW

AC is largely a diagnosis of exclusion based on the patient's history, physical examination, and ruling out other etiologies of a painful shoulder (arthritis, rotator cuff or labral tear, radiculopathy). A detailed discussion of risk factors which may raise clinical suspicion is provided below. Generally, in AC, patients tend to present with several months of shoulder pain before they experience the loss of ROM.[6,10] Commonly, this pain localizes to the origin of the deltoid muscle and may be associated with night pain; patients may not be able to sleep on the affected side. Of note, pain with overhead motion is more suggestive of other shoulder pathology and is not often seen in AC.[10]

As AC progresses (see stages below), patients begin to lose ROM in the affected shoulder, first with the loss of internal and/or external rotation; often, they have difficulty performing activities of daily living such as dressing, brushing their hair, or reaching their back pocket. Eventually, almost all ROM (including passive) is lost, and pain begins to decrease. This painless loss of motion is evident only in the later stages of AC and is limited by the contracted joint capsule.[6,10]

On physical examination, patients tend to lack focal tenderness to palpation, other than over the biceps tendon because its synovium communicates with that of the GH joint. However, sometimes there is tenderness at the rotator interval (RI), just lateral to the coracoid, although this can be a nonspecific finding. Passive ROM is limited by a firm endpoint or mechanical block, which is essentially diagnostic of AC. In particular, internal/external rotation and forward elevation are commonly limited on examination. Patients may experience pain only when the shoulder is taken through extremes of motion, beyond what the contracted joint capsule would allow.[6,10]

The diagnosis of AC is primarily made clinically, and radiographs of the shoulder are usually normal in this disease process, the only exception being in patients who develop disuse osteopenia from chronic disease. However, there is still utility in ordering plain films to rule out other causes of shoulder pain (arthritis, calcific tendinitis, and so forth). Although MRI, magnetic resonance arthrogram (MRA), and ultrasound are not primary diagnostic tools, there are certain findings that may confirm a diagnosis of AC (**Fig. 1**). These include thickening of the joint capsule or coracohumeral ligament (CHL), loss of the axillary recess, joint capsule edema, loss of subcoracoid fat, or hypervascularity of the joint capsule.[6,10-12]

Risk Factors

Although the prevalence of AC is 2% to 5%, it occurs most commonly in women (up to 70% of all cases), between the ages of 40 and 60, in patients with diabetes mellitus (DM), and is bilateral in up to 25% of patients.[6,11,13] Other established risk factors include previous surgery (shoulder, breast cancer, or cervical spine), thyroid disease, cardiac disease, HLA-B27 positivity, Dupuytren's disease, rarely immunizations (pneumococcal), and even COVID-19.[6,11,13-20]

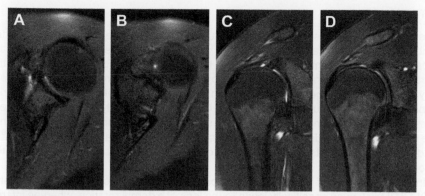

Fig. 1. MRI findings of adhesive capsulitis. Note the thickened capsule and relative lack of subcoracoid fat on the axial images (*A, B*) and lack of axillary recess on coronal images (*C, D*).

Diabetes Mellitus

A recent meta-analysis of 18 studies found the overall mean prevalence of AC in a population of DM to be 13.4%.[21] Conversely, the mean prevalence of DM in a population of AC was 30%, and patients with DM (compared with those without) were five times more likely to develop AC. In addition, patients with DM tend to get AC at a younger age than non-diabetics, and the incidence of AC correlates with how long someone has been diabetic.[12] Interestingly, there does not seem to be a correlation between hemoglobin A_{1c} level and AC prevalence.[22,23] Finally, it remains uncertain whether there is a significant difference in AC prevalence in DM1 versus DM2, or insulin-dependence versus other therapies.[21,22]

Previous Surgery

There have been many studies that have examined the relationship between recent shoulder surgery and the prevalence of AC. Although the prevalence ranges from 5% to 11%,[11] a recent prospective cohort study found that 11% of patients at 6 months follow-up from elective shoulder surgery developed AC, which was more common in women (15%) versus men (8%).[15] After breast cancer surgery, the prevalence of AC is about 10% and higher in those who undergo mastectomy rather than lumpectomy.[19] After cervical disk surgery, patients have 1.66 times higher risk for developing AC at 6 months follow-up compared with control.[18]

Thyroid Disease

Huang and colleagues performed a 7-year prospective study including one million patients and found that patients with hyperthyroidism had a hazard ratio of 1.22 (95% confidence interval [CI], 1.03–1.45) when compared with the control group for developing AC.[24] Thus, hyperthyroidism is considered an independent risk factor for the development of AC. Hypothyroidism has also been associated with AC.[6]

COVID-19

Finally, a case series was recently published of 12 patients who developed AC after COVID-19.[14]

PATHOANATOMY

The RI is the triangular space in the anterosuperior aspect of the GH joint that provides stability to the GH joint and biceps tendon.[25] The RI contains the CHL, long head of the biceps tendon, and joint capsule. The RI is bordered medially (base of triangle) by the coracoid process, laterally (tip of triangle) by the transverse humeral ligament, superiorly by the anterior aspect of the supraspinatus tendon, and inferiorly by the superior aspect of the subscapularis tendon.[25] The CHL, which normally is composed of flexible Type 3 collagen, originates from the base of the coracoid process and inserts into the RI, acting as a "holder" for both the subscapularis and supraspinatus muscles.[26] In addition, the CHL limits external rotation of the shoulder to provide stability to the shoulder joint.[27]

In AC, contraction of the RI and joint capsule results in a loss of active and passive ROM.[6] RI thickening specifically leads to the loss of external rotation, whereas inferior capsular thickening leads to the loss of elevation and posterior capsular thickening leads to the loss of internal rotation. Other pathoanatomic findings in AC are a thicker capsule, smaller volume of the axillary recess, loss of subcoracoid fat, and distention of the subscapularis bursa.[6,27] Most importantly, the CHL is contracted, thickened, and stiffened when compared with healthy shoulders which subsequently limits external rotation.[6,27]

PATHOGENESIS

The pathogenesis of AC is not entirely understood and is most often idiopathic. However, it generally begins as an inflammatory reaction involving cytokines (transforming growth factor beta, tumor necrosis factor alpha, cyclooxygenase [COX-1 and COX-2], and interleukins [IL]) and leukocytes (B- and T-lymphocytes, macrophages, and mast cells).[6,11,28] After this inflammatory phase, a fibrotic phase ensues which involves fibroblasts mixed with type I and type III collagen, histologic findings similar to those seen in Dupuytren's disease.[6] Specifically, these fibroblasts transform into myofibroblasts which may be responsible for GH joint capsule and RI contracture.[6] In addition, there is an imbalance between matrix melloproteinases (MMPs), involved in scar tissue remodeling and collagen degradation, and tissue inhibitor of metalloproteinases (TIMPs). Thus, there is an imbalance in extracellular matrix remodeling favoring excess fibrogenesis and fibrosis.[6,29]

There may also be a genetic predisposition to the MMP/TIMP imbalance seen in AC. In their cytogenetic analysis of AC synovium, Kabbabe and colleagues demonstrated elevated levels of MMP-3 and IL-6 (inflammatory cytokines) when compared with controls.[29] Subsequently, Ling and colleagues characterized single nuclear polymorphisms of both MMP-3 and IL-6 which were associated with increased risk for severity of post-operative shoulder stiffness.[30]

Four stages of AC have been described based on the arthroscopic and histologic appearance of the joint capsule, from inflammation to fibrosis.[10] In stage 1, the preadhesive stage, there is fibrinous inflammation of the synovium without adhesions. Patients have full ROM but may have night pain. In stage 2, adhesions begin to form, mostly in the inferior capsular fold. Patients begin to lose some ROM, but pain is the most severe during this stage. During stage 3, the maturation stage, inflammation begins to decrease, and fibrosis of the capsule begins. Patients now have a significant loss of ROM, but pain begins to improve. Finally, in stage 4, the chronic stage, adhesions are matured and there is a significant, painless loss of ROM.

NATURAL HISTORY AND NONOPERATIVE TREATMENT

The literature on the natural history of AC is relatively limited and the outcome of idiopathic frozen shoulder remains somewhat controversial. Neviaser and Neviaser classically described the four stages of AC, as noted above: Stage I: shoulder pain, primarily at night, with perseveration of motion; Stage 2: development of stiffness; Stage 3: profound global loss of ROM and pain at extremes of ROM; Stage 4: persistent stiffness with improvement of pain.[31] The stages have also been summarized as the "painful phase," "stiff phase," and "thawing phase."

When it comes to the reported outcomes of untreated or nonoperatively treated frozen shoulders, the data have been somewhat mixed. Reeve's prospective study of 41 patients treated nonoperatively found that only 39% regained full shoulder ROM at 5 to 10 years.[32] Other studies, however, have reported 89% to 100% of patients regaining complete or near complete restoration of shoulder ROM after nonoperative treatment.[33–35] Diercks and Stevens reported in their prospective study of 45 patients that 89% achieved Constant–Murley scores of 80 or greater.[35] The shortest mean duration of idiopathic AC without treatment has been reported at 15 months,[35,36] and the longest mean duration has been 30 months.[32] Overall, the literature suggests that the natural history is largely benign, which matches with the author's clinical experience.

In a more recent and robust review of the natural history of idiopathic frozen shoulder with a 2- to 27-year follow-up (mean, 9 years), Vastamäki and colleagues followed 83 patients having undergone either observation/benign neglect (51 patients) or nonoperative treatment (32). The authors found that untreated group had a mean duration of disease of 15 months compared with 20 months in the nonoperatively treated group. At final follow-up, the shoulder ROM had been restored to that of the contralateral shoulder in 91% to 94% of patients. Resolution of pain, however, did not improve as much as ROM did. The authors found that only 44% to 51% of patients achieved complete resolution of pain at rest, during the night, and with activity at the time of final follow-up. However, visual analog scaleVAS) scores were less than 3 in 91% to 94% of patients. Their patients were able to reach what would be the expected for normal age and gender-related Constant–Murley scores.[36] Generally, based on the conducted research on idiopathic ACs natural history, it can be said with a relatively high degree of confidence that patients will recover without restriction of motion or pain.

Nonoperative Treatment Options

As frustrating as AC is to the patient and their doctor, it may well be a self-limiting phenomenon. Thus, the treatment strategies vary considerably, from benign neglect to invasive open surgical procedures. Treatments are often geared toward the specific phase of AC. Oral anti-inflammatory medications (NSAIDs), physical therapy, and injections are often used in the first two phases of AC. Medications and injections can be helpful in reducing pain enough to make physical therapy tolerable. There is no universally accepted treatment algorithm and doctors must work together with their patients to create a plan. Nonoperative management with the above measures results in satisfactory outcomes in 60% to 90% of cases.[33,37]

Physical Therapy

Early mobilization and physical therapy are often used as first-line treatments for AC. Protocols vary and physical therapy is frequently typically combined with other modalities to give the greatest benefit. Generally, there is support for the use of physical therapy in the literature, but how aggressive one should be with therapy remains controversial. Vermeulen and colleagues showed only small differences in outcome between gentle (low grade) and aggressive (high-grade) mobilization therapy at 1 year, slightly favoring high-grade therapy.[38] Another prospective study comparing pendulum and gentle exercises (supervised neglect) vs intensive physical therapy demonstrated better results with gentle exercises at 2-year follow-up, with 89% of gentle exercise group as opposed to 63% of the intensive therapy group achieving normal or near-normal painless shoulder function.[35] Although early mobilization is generally recommended, if patients are in the initial "painful phase," aggressive therapy may not be tolerable. As such, some clinicians wait until their patients are out of the "painful phase" before initiating physical therapy or recommend only gentle exercises at first. This approach is supported by the findings Griggs and colleagues, who demonstrated that waiting until patients are in the "stiffness phase" still resulted in 90% satisfactory outcomes.[33] Alternatively, providing a cortisone injection before initiating therapy can provide a better experience for both the patient and the therapist.

Home exercise programs may be equally effective as supervised therapy[39] and with growing interest in telehealth, there is a multicenter randomized controlled trial underway that is evaluating telerehabilitation for patients with AC.[40] Overall, a recent systematic review of various physical therapy protocols concluded that there is inadequate evidence at this time to determine the superiority of one modality versus another, and thus adequately sampled randomized controlled trials are likely necessary to make that determination.[41]

Corticosteroid Injections

Intra-articular corticosteroid injections seem to be effective in the early stages of AC. In their retrospective study, Ahn and colleagues found that injection earlier in the disease course seemed shorten the duration of symptoms.[42] In their study, patients received an ultrasound-guided steroid injection after at least 1 month of unsuccessful conservative treatment. Outcomes at 1 and 12 months after injection were better the earlier they had received the injection in their disease course. Prestgaard and colleagues performed a double-blind, placebo-controlled randomized study that demonstrated a significant decrease in shoulder pain at 6 and 12 weeks in those receiving ultrasound-guided intra-articular and RI steroid injections.[43] These results were no longer notable at 26 weeks. According to Raeissadat and colleagues, ultrasound-guidance seems to improve pain, ROM, and functional scores compared with blind intra-articular injection technique, though statistically significant differences were not found.[44] Compared with physical therapy alone, corticosteroid injections alone do not seem to provide a significant benefit, according to a 2016 metanalysis.[45] However, corticosteroid injections used in conjunction with physical therapy, seem to improve symptoms better than physical therapy alone, at least in the short term.[46] A recent meta-analysis of placebo controlled and comparative studies found a significant short-term clinical advantage of steroid injections over placebo.[47] In addition, the meta-analysis found that ultrasound-guided RI injections and multiple-site injections seem to improve outcomes at intermediate term (2–6 months).[47]

Hydrodistension

Hydrodistension involves injection of fluid under image-guidance, either fluoroscopic or ultrasonographic, to stretch the contracted capsule, thereby increasing intracapsular volume of the GH joint. It is most frequently performed in refractory cases and can be performed with joint manipulation under interscalene block at the time of hydrodistension.[48] Multiple studies have shown short-term benefit of hydrodistension with or without simultaneous intra-articular steroid injection, but this effect seems to diminish by the 1-year mark.[48,49] One randomized controlled trial, however, did not show a treatment benefit of hydrodistension with corticosteroid compared with corticosteroid injection alone.[50]

Hyaluronic Acid

Hyaluronic acid (HA) is an integral part of the synovial fluid, responsible for joint lubrication and chondroprotection. Intra-articular HA injection reduces cytokine-induced responses and reduces synovial inflammation, which can alleviate pain and improve function.[51] Its utility in AC remains controversial. Although some have reported improvements with HA injections combined with physical therapy,[52] a systemic review of four RCTs found no difference in shoulder functional outcomes or pain when comparing HA with conventional therapy.[53]

Collagenase

There has been recent interest in the use of collagenase for AC. Collagenase is a degradative enzyme isolated from the bacterium Clostridium histolyticum. It has been approved for the treatment of Dupuytren's disease and Peyronie's disease, two fibrotic tissue disorders with histologic similarities to AC. A placebo-controlled double-blind RCT found improvement in motion, pain, and function with collagenase injection compared with exercise alone at short-term follow-up.[54] Others have not found significant improvements and have reported on the adverse effects, namely local tenderness and bruising, with bruising ranging from localized around the injection site, to entire upper arm and chest wall.[55]

Other Nonoperative Therapies

Suprascapular nerve blocks are commonly used perioperatively for shoulder surgery patients. The suprascapular nerve provides sensory fibers to approximately 70% of the GH joint and guided injections of the nerve seem to be a feasible option for patients, particularly those whose symptoms have been refractory to intra-articular steroid injections.[56]

Extracorporeal shock wave therapy (ECSWT) has been investigated for the treatment of AC. One randomized controlled trial of 40 patients treated with either ECSWT or oral steroids demonstrated improvement in Constant Shoulder Score and ROM at 4 weeks and (activities of daily living) ADL function at 6 weeks in patient treated with ECSWT.[57] It has also been shown to improve functional outcomes in diabetic patients and therefore may be preferable to oral or injected corticosteroids in this subset of patients to mitigate the impact of those preparations on blood glucose levels.[58]

Calcitonin is a polypeptide hormone secreted from the parafollicular cells of the thyroid and has been used as an analgesic augment in various musculoskeletal conditions, including complex regional pain syndrome, rheumatoid arthritis, and bone tumors. Its mechanism of action is not entirely understood, but it is thought to work by decreasing systemic inflammation and stimulating endorphin release. A double-blinded randomized controlled trial of 64 patients with AC demonstrated improvement in shoulder pain, ROM, and functional scores at 6 weeks after treatment with intranasal calcitonin compared with the placebo group.[59] This may be another useful modality in the physician's toolbox for managing AC-related pain.

SURGICAL TREATMENT OPTIONS

After 9 to 12 months of inadequate symptom relief with nonsurgical therapies including NSAIDs, PT, injections, and the other modalities described above, the orthopedic surgeon may consider operative intervention. The options include manipulation under anesthesia (MUA), arthroscopic capsular release, and open capsular release.

Manipulation Under Anesthesia

The general idea of MUA is to stretch the contracted shoulder capsule beyond the patient's normal pain thresholds. It is a relatively safe procedure, but complications such as hemarthrosis, labral tears, and even humeral and glenoid fractures have been described.[6] In addition, the results of MUA are mixed. Multiple studies have found equivalent or even decreased symptomatic and functional improvements in patients treated with MUA compared with PT, home exercises, or steroid injections.[60–62] Recurrent frozen shoulder after MUA is also a recognized entity. In their prospective study, Woods and colleagues performed repeat MUA in 18% of 792 shoulders. Patients with type-1 DM were at 38% increased risk of requiring further MUA.[63] It is for the reasons listed above that MUA alone, without arthroscopic capsular release, is not generally encouraged.

Arthroscopic Capsular Release

Open capsulotomy has essentially been replaced by arthroscopic techniques because of the improved visualization, shorter recovery time, and the less invasive nature of arthroscopy. Arthroscopic capsular release has been demonstrated in multiple studies to be an effective in the treatment of refractory primary and secondary AC, with minimal complications.[64–70] It allows the surgeon to perform diagnostic arthroscopy to rule out other pathologies within the shoulder and also allows direct visualization of the thickened RI, contracted capsule, and tightened CHL. There are various techniques to perform an arthroscopic capsular release and there is no consensus regarding the optimal extent of capsular release. Some surgeons perform circumferential release,[67,69,70] whereas others prefer limited anterior releases.[71,72] In addition to the improvement of external rotation and elevation with anterior-inferior releases, a posterior capsular release has been described to improve internal rotation.[73,74]

Overall success rates of arthroscopic release are above 80% in the non-diabetic population,[67,75] but diabetic patients are reported to have more residual pain, reduced motion and function, and need for revision surgery.[76] A systematic review by Boutefnouchet and colleagues demonstrated that 26% of diabetic patients had recurrent pain and 8.1% had revision surgery, compared with 0% and 2.4%, respectively, in patients with idiopathic AC.[76]

Although risk of axillary nerve injury is very low with all techniques, it should be known that the axillary nerve runs nearer to the humeral insertion than to the glenoid insertion of the joint capsule. It is therefore safer to position the arm in abduction when performing the inferior release, as this will increase the distance between the axillary nerve and the joint capsule.[77] Alternatively, the surgeon should consider lateral decubitus positioning with the arm in traction to arthroscopic release the inferior capsule as this position provides better visualization of the inferior capsule.

A retrospective review of 56 shoulders treated with circumferential release demonstrated significant improvements in shoulder ROM (mean elevation and external rotation increases of 45° and 41°, respectively) and shoulder pain at a mean of 65 months.[69] Lafosse and colleagues prospectively evaluated 10 patients treated with circumferential arthroscopic releases and also found significant improvements in pain, ROM, and functional outcomes at an average of 42 month follow-up, without any complications.[70]

A recent systematic review and meta-analysis of 18 studies comparing anterior-inferior capsular release vs anterior-inferior-posterior capsular release vs circumferential capsular release suggests that less extensive releases may actually result in better functional and pain scores. The authors suggest that posterior release offers increased internal rotation early on, but this is not sustained over time, and that a circumferential release may not provide any further benefit. Also, there were no significant differences in complications among the techniques.[68] The randomized controlled trial by Kim and colleagues demonstrated no benefit of adding a posterior release to anterior release, citing no significant differences in functional scores, pain, or postoperative ROM in all planes.[72]

A general anesthetic with paralysis ensures that after capsular release is performed, gentle examination under anesthesia can be accomplished to ensure that ROM is restored. Regardless of extent of capsular release, it is beneficial to have the anesthesiologist perform an interscalene block with a continuous catheter to deliver prolonged analgesia in the postoperative period.[11,78] This enables the patient to perform active and passive ROM of the shoulder in the days following surgery. Multimodal pain management is integral to the recovery process and helps to reduce narcotic usage. Postoperative medications may include scheduled acetaminophen and gabapentin, diazepam as needed for muscle spasm, and then an oral narcotic as needed for severe pain.

Physical therapy should begin as soon as possible after surgery, and this goal is achieved with the help of anesthetic blocks and/or continues pain catheters, as described above. Physical therapy (PT) should focus on achieving a functional ROM. Our post-op PT protocol involves immediate and aggressive passive ROM and capsular mobility in all planes three to four times per day, scapular mobility exercises initiated immediately, and active ROM as tolerated. We recommend patients be supervised by a therapist three times per week in the first several weeks to ensure ROM is improving. A sling is used only for comfort. We also recommend heat before and ice after therapy sessions. At 6 weeks post-op, patients begin strengthening as tolerated.

Although complication rates after simultaneous arthroscopic capsular release and MUA are low, complications such as iatrogenic labral tears, humeral and glenoid fractures, axillary nerve injury, shoulder dislocations, and complex regional pain syndrome have been reported.[6,79] In addition, in the small percentage of patients who have continued frozen shoulder after surgery, repeat arthroscopy and MUA is likely to be successful.[63]

The senior author's preferred surgical technique for arthroscopic capsular release is as follows. The patient is positioned in the beach chair position. First, the shoulder is manipulated into passive forward elevation. This maneuver will tear the inferior capsule, and thus the surgeon does not need to perform an inferior capsular release, and thus the surgeon can avoid any potential injury to the axillary nerve. In addition, this provides a greater ability to distract the humerus from the glenoid during trocar insertion, thus reducing the risk for chondral injury during entry. Then, a posterior viewing portal and anterosuperior working portals are established. Through the anterosuperior portal, the RI capsule is released with a radiofrequency ablation wand until the coracoacromial ligament can be visualized. This release is then continued inferiorly

- MUA into passive forward elevation
- Scope from posterior and release interval capsule until CA can be seen
- Continue capsular release anterior to subscapularis until you get to 5 o'clock/ruptured capsule
- Scope from anterior and release posterior capsule from portal inferior until you get to 7 o'clock/ruptured capsule

Fig. 2. Senior author's key surgical steps.

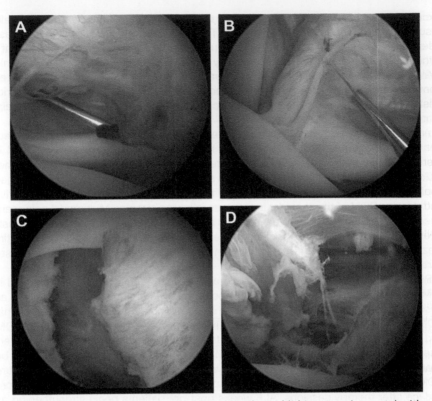

Fig. 3. Arthroscopic images of capsular release (*A, B*). Establishing anterior portal with spinal needle, noting increased capsular thickness. (*C*) Anterior release viewing from posterior portal. (*D*) Posterior release viewing from anterior portal.

along the posterior aspect of the subscapularis until the tear in the inferior capsule is encountered or the 5 o'clock position is reached, whichever comes first. The arthroscope and instruments are then withdrawn, and then, it is confirmed that full passive external rotation can be achieved. This is an examination under anesthesia and not an MUA as the anterior capsule has been completely released. Of note, an external rotation MUA is the maneuver that creates the greatest risk for fracture and thus should be avoided. The arthroscope is then inserted into the anterosuperior portal, and the radiofrequency ablation wand is inserted into the posterior portal. The posterior capsule is then released, again until the inferior capsular tear is encountered or the 7 o'clock position is reached, whichever comes first. If is then confirmed that full internal rotation can be achieved, again as an examination under anesthesia and not an MUA. This sequence of steps avoids most of the significant risks (axillary nerve injury, intraoperative fracture) traditionally associated with the procedure, provides a circumferential release, and can be rapidly performed in the beach chair position. The main surgical steps are summarized in **Fig. 2**, and arthroscopic images are depicted in **Fig. 3**.

SUMMARY

AC is a relatively common orthopedic condition, affecting up to 5% of the population and occurring more frequently in women, patients with diabetes or thyroid disease, and those having undergone recent surgery. It generally begins as an inflammatory reaction and a resultant imbalance in extracellular matrix remodeling favoring excess fibrogenesis and fibrosis. This leads to extensive scar tissue formation and contracture of the capsule, with associated pain and stiffness that occur in four classic stages of the disease. It seems that an early intervention with corticosteroid injection, NSAIDs, and physical therapy have a role in shortening the duration of the disease. Other nonoperative options exist and may provide benefit. There has been recent interest in the use of collagenase injections for treating AC, but more data are needed regarding its efficacy. Patients should know that a vast majority of cases resolve with nonoperative management. However, in cases refractory to the above nonoperative measures, there is a role for surgery. Arthroscopic capsular release, ranging from anteroinferior to circumferential release, with gentle MUA has a very high success rate (>80%), though diabetic patients have poorer outcomes compared with those with idiopathic AC. Complication rates are very low with surgery, and postoperative pain control is essential to allow for physical therapy early in the recovery process.

CLINICS CARE POINTS

Pearls
- Risk factors for adhesive capsulitis (AC) include diabetes, thyroid disease, recent surgery, and perhaps COVID-19 infection.
- Limited shoulder active and passive ROM, particularly external rotation and forward elevation, should raise suspicion for AC.
- Treatment with NSAIDs, corticosteroid injection, and physical therapy should be implemented early in the disease process and this may shorten duration of symptoms.
- When nonoperative treatment fails, arthroscopic capsular release is a highly successful treatment option.

Pitfalls
- Delay in diagnosis and initiation of early treatment may lead to a prolonged clinical course and/or need for arthroscopic capsular release.
- Complications of arthroscopic capsular release and manipulation under anesthesia include iatrogenic labral tears, humeral and glenoid fractures, and axillary nerve injury, so care must be exercised during these operations.
- Delayed initiation or noncompliance with postoperative PT may diminish the results after arthroscopic capsular release.

DISCLOSURE

The authors have nothing to disclose.

REFERENCES

1. Mäkelä M, Heliövaara M, Sainio P, et al. Shoulder joint impairment among Finns aged 30 years or over: prevalence, risk factors and co-morbidity. Rheumatology (Oxford, England) 1999;38(7). https://doi.org/10.1093/rheumatology/38.7.656.
2. Huang SW, Lin JW, Wang WT, et al. Hyperthyroidism is a risk factor for developing adhesive capsulitis of the shoulder: a nationwide longitudinal population-based study. Scientific Rep 2014;4. https://doi.org/10.1038/srep04183.
3. Neviaser AS, Neviaser RJ. Adhesive capsulitis of the shoulder. J Am Acad Orthopaedic Surgeons 2011;19(9). https://doi.org/10.5435/00124635-201109000-00004.
4. D'Orsi GM, Via AG, Frizziero A, et al. Treatment of adhesive capsulitis: a review. Muscles, ligaments tendons J 2012;2(2).

5. Neviaser JS. Adhesive capsulitis of the shoulder: a study of the pathological findings in periarthritis of the shoulder. J Bone Joint Surg 1945;27(2):211–22.
6. Le H v, Lee SJ, Nazarian A, et al. Adhesive capsulitis of the shoulder: review of pathophysiology and current clinical treatments. Shoulder Elbow 2017;9(2): 75–84.
7. Binder AI, Bulgen DY, Hazleman BL, et al. Frozen shoulder: a long-term prospective study. Ann Rheum Dis 1984;43(3). https://doi.org/10.1136/ard.43.3.361.
8. Shaffer B, Tibone JE, Kerlan RK. Frozen shoulder. a long-term follow-up. J bone Jt Surg Am volume 1992;74(5).
9. Hand C, Clipsham K, Rees JL, et al. Long-term outcome of frozen shoulder. J Shoulder Elbow Surg 2008;17(2). https://doi.org/10.1016/j.jse.2007.05.009.
10. Neviaser AS, Neviaser RJ. Adhesive capsulitis of the shoulder. Am Acad Orthopaedic Surgeon 2011;19(9). https://doi.org/10.5435/00124635-201109000-00004.
11. Redler LH, Dennis ER. Treatment of adhesive capsulitis of the shoulder. J Am Acad Orthopaedic Surgeons 2019;27(12):E544–54.
12. Santoboni F, Balducci S, DErrico V, et al. Extracorporeal shockwave therapy improves functional outcomes of adhesive capsulitis of the shoulder in patients with diabetes. Diabetes Care 2017;40(2):e12–3. https://doi.org/10.2337/dc16-2063.
13. Georgiannos D, Markopoulos G, Devetzi E, et al. Adhesive capsulitis of the shoulder. is there consensus regarding the treatment? a comprehensive review. Open Orthopaedics J 2017;11(1). https://doi.org/10.2174/1874325001711010065.
14. Ascani C, Passaretti D, Scacchi M, et al. Can adhesive capsulitis of the shoulder be a consequence of COVID-19? Case series of 12 patients. J Shoulder Elbow Surg 2021;30(7). https://doi.org/10.1016/j.jse.2021.04.024.
15. Koorevaar RCT, vant-Riet E, Ipskamp M, et al. Incidence and prognostic factors for postoperative frozen shoulder after shoulder surgery: a prospective cohort study. Arch Orthop Trauma Surg 2017;137(3). https://doi.org/10.1007/s00402-016-2589-3.
16. Denard PJ, Lädermann A, Burkhart SS. Prevention and management of stiffness after arthroscopic rotator cuff repair: Systematic review and implications for rotator cuff healing. Arthrosc - J Arthroscopic Relat Surg 2011;27(6). https://doi.org/10.1016/j.arthro.2011.01.013.
17. Saleh ZM, Faruqui S, Foad A. Onset of frozen shoulder following pneumococcal and influenza vaccinations. J Chiropractic Med 2015;14(4). https://doi.org/10.1016/j.jcm.2015.05.005.
18. Kang JH, Lin HC, Tsai MC, et al. Increased risk for adhesive capsulitis of the shoulder following cervical disc surgery. Scientific Rep 2016;6. https://doi.org/10.1038/srep26898.
19. Yang S, Park DH, Ahn SH, et al. Prevalence and risk factors of adhesive capsulitis of the shoulder after breast cancer treatment. Support Care Cancer 2017;25(4). https://doi.org/10.1007/s00520-016-3532-4.
20. Evans JP, Guyver PM, Smith CD. Frozen shoulder after simple arthroscopic shoulder procedures: What is the risk? Bone Joint J 2015;97-B(7). https://doi.org/10.1302/0301-620X.97B7.35387.
21. Zreik NH, Malik RA, Charalambous CP. Adhesive capsulitis of the shoulder and diabetes: a meta-analysis of prevalence. Muscles Ligaments Tendons J 2019; 6(1):26–34. https://doi.org/10.11138/mltj/2016.6.1.026.
22. Yian EH, Contreras R, Sodl JF. Effects of glycemic control on prevalence of diabetic frozen shoulder. J Bone Joint Surg - Ser A 2012;94(10):919–23. https://doi.org/10.2106/JBJS.J.01930.

23. Thomas SJ, McDougall C, Brown IDM, et al. Prevalence of symptoms and signs of shoulder problems in people with diabetes mellitus. J Shoulder Elbow Surg 2007;16(6):748–51. https://doi.org/10.1016/j.jse.2007.02.133.

24. Huang SW, Lin JW, Wang WT, et al. Hyperthyroidism is a risk factor for developing adhesive capsulitis of the shoulder: a nationwide longitudinal population-based study. Sci Rep 2014;4:4183. Available at: www.nature.com/scientificreports.

25. Hunt SA, Kwon YW, Zuckerman JD. The rotator interval: anatomy, pathology, and strategies for treatment. J Am Acad Orthopaedic Surgeons 2007;15(4). https://doi.org/10.5435/00124635-200704000-00005.

26. Arai R, Nimura A, Yamaguchi K, et al. The anatomy of the coracohumeral ligament and its relation to the subscapularis muscle. J Shoulder Elbow Surg 2014;23(10). https://doi.org/10.1016/j.jse.2014.02.009.

27. McKean D, Chung SL, te Water Naudé R, et al. Elasticity of the coracohumeral ligament in patients with frozen shoulder following rotator interval injection: a case series. J Ultrasonography 2020;20(83). https://doi.org/10.15557/JoU.2020.0052.

28. Lho YM, Ha E, Cho CH, et al. Inflammatory cytokines are overexpressed in the subacromial bursa of frozen shoulder. J Shoulder Elbow Surg 2013;22(5). https://doi.org/10.1016/j.jse.2012.06.014.

29. Kabbabe B, Ramkumar S, Richardson M. Cytogenetic analysis of the pathology of frozen shoulder. Int J Shoulder Surg 2010;4(3). https://doi.org/10.4103/0973-6042.76966.

30. Ling Y, Peng C, Liu C, et al. Gene polymorphism of IL-6 and MMP-3 decreases passive range of motion after rotator cuff repair. Int J Clin Exp Pathol 2015;8(5).

31. Neviaser RJ, Neviaser TJ. The frozen shoulder. diagnosis and management. Clin Orthopaedics Relat Res 1987;223:59–64.

32. Reeves B. The natural history of the frozen shoulder syndrome. Scand J Rheumatol 1975;4(4). https://doi.org/10.3109/03009747509165255.

33. Griggs SM, Ahn A, Green A. Idiopathic adhesive capsulitis. A prospective functional outcome study of nonoperative treatment. J bone Jt Surg Am volume 2000;82(10).

34. Dudkiewicz I, Oran A, Salai M, et al. Idiopathic adhesive capsulitis: long-term results of conservative treatment. Isr Med Assoc J : IMAJ 2004;6(9):524–6.

35. Diercks RL, Stevens M. Gentle thawing of the frozen shoulder: a prospective study of supervised neglect versus intensive physical therapy in seventy-seven patients with frozen shoulder syndrome followed up for two years. J Shoulder Elbow Surg 2004;13(5). https://doi.org/10.1016/j.jse.2004.03.002.

36. Vastamäki H, Kettunen J, Vastamäki M. The natural history of idiopathic frozen shoulder: a 2- to 27-year followup study. Clin orthopaedics Relat Res 2012;470(4). https://doi.org/10.1007/s11999-011-2176-4.

37. Wallny T, Melzer C, Wagner U, et al. ["Primary" shoulder stiffness: illness duration and therapeutic comparison]. Z Orthopadie ihre Grenzgebiete 1997;135(3). https://doi.org/10.1055/s-2008-1039584.

38. Vermeulen HM, Rozing PM, Obermann WR, et al. Comparison of high-grade and low-grade mobilization techniques in the management of adhesive capsulitis of the shoulder: randomized controlled trial. Phys Ther 2006;86(3).

39. Tanaka K, Saura R, Takahashi N, et al. Joint mobilization versus self-exercises for limited glenohumeral joint mobility: randomized controlled study of management of rehabilitation. Clin Rheumatol 2010;29(12). https://doi.org/10.1007/s10067-010-1525-0.

40. Yeo SM, Lim JY, Do JG, Lim JY, Lee J, Hwang JH. Effectiveness of interactive augmented reality-based telerehabilitation in patients with adhesive capsulitis: protocol for a multi-center randomized controlled trial. BMC Musculoskelet Disord 2021;22(1). https://doi.org/10.1186/s12891-021-04261-1.

41. Nakandala P, Nanayakkara I, Wadugodapitiya S, et al. The efficacy of physiotherapy interventions in the treatment of adhesive capsulitis: A systematic review. J Back Musculoskelet Rehabil 2021;34(2). https://doi.org/10.3233/BMR-200186.

42. Ahn JH, Lee DH, Kang H, et al. Early intra-articular corticosteroid injection improves pain and function in adhesive capsulitis of the shoulder: 1-year retrospective longitudinal study. PM R : Journal Injury, Function, Rehabilitation 2018;10(1). https://doi.org/10.1016/j.pmrj.2017.06.004.

43. Prestgaard T, Wormgoor MEA, Haugen S, et al. Ultrasound-guided intra-articular and rotator interval corticosteroid injections in adhesive capsulitis of the shoulder: a double-blind, sham-controlled randomized study. Pain 2015;156(9). https://doi.org/10.1097/j.pain.0000000000000209.

44. Raeissadat SA, Rayegani SM, Langroudi TF, et al. Comparing the accuracy and efficacy of ultrasound-guided versus blind injections of steroid in the glenohumeral joint in patients with shoulder adhesive capsulitis. Clin Rheumatol 2017;36(4). https://doi.org/10.1007/s10067-016-3393-8.

45. Sun Y, Lu S, Zhang P, et al. Steroid injection versus physiotherapy for patients with adhesive capsulitis of the shoulder: a PRIMSA systematic review and meta-analysis of randomized controlled trials. Medicine 2016;95(20). https://doi.org/10.1097/MD.0000000000003469.

46. Sharma SP, Bærheim A, Moe-Nilssen R, et al. Adhesive capsulitis of the shoulder, treatment with corticosteroid, corticosteroid with distension or treatment-as-usual; a randomised controlled trial in primary care. BMC Musculoskelet Disord 2016; 17. https://doi.org/10.1186/s12891-016-1081-0.

47. Kitridis D, Tsikopoulos K, Bisbinas I, et al. Efficacy of pharmacological therapies for adhesive capsulitis of the shoulder: a systematic review and network meta-analysis. Am J Sports Med 2019;47(14). https://doi.org/10.1177/0363546518823337.

48. Mun SW, Baek CH. Clinical efficacy of hydrodistention with joint manipulation under interscalene block compared with intra-articular corticosteroid injection for frozen shoulder: a prospective randomized controlled study. J Shoulder Elbow Surg 2016;25(12). https://doi.org/10.1016/j.jse.2016.09.021.

49. Yoong P, Duffy S, McKean D, et al. Targeted ultrasound-guided hydrodilatation via the rotator interval for adhesive capsulitis. Skeletal Radiol 2015;44(5). https://doi.org/10.1007/s00256-014-2047-7.

50. Lee DH, Yoon SH, Lee MY, et al. Capsule-preserving hydrodilatation with corticosteroid versus corticosteroid injection alone in refractory adhesive capsulitis of shoulder: a randomized controlled trial. Arch Phys Med Rehabil 2017;98(5). https://doi.org/10.1016/j.apmr.2016.10.012.

51. Iwata H. Pharmacologic and clinical aspects of intraarticular injection of hyaluronate. Clin Orthopaedics Relat Res 1993;289:285–91.

52. Russo A, Arrighi A, Vignale L, et al. Conservative integrated treatment of adhesive capsulitis of the shoulder. Joints 2014;2(1):15–9.

53. Lee LC, Lieu FK, Lee HL, et al. Effectiveness of hyaluronic acid administration in treating adhesive capsulitis of the shoulder: a systematic review of randomized controlled trials. Biomed Research International 2015;2015. https://doi.org/10.1155/2015/314120.

54. Badalamente MA, Wang ED. CORR® ORS richard a. brand award: clinical trials of a new treatment Method for Adhesive Capsulitis. Clin Orthopaedics Relat Res 2016;474(11). https://doi.org/10.1007/s11999-016-4862-8.
55. Fitzpatrick J, Richardson C, Klaber I, et al. Clostridium histolyticum (AA4500) for the treatment of adhesive capsulitis of the shoulder: a randomised double-blind, placebo-controlled study for the safety and efficacy of collagenase - single site report. Drug Des Dev Ther 2020;14. https://doi.org/10.2147/DDDT.S259228.
56. Ozkan K, Ozcekic AN, Sarar S, et al. Suprascapular nerve block for the treatment of frozen shoulder. Saudi J Anaesth 2012;6(1). https://doi.org/10.4103/1658-354X.93061.
57. Chen CY, Hu CC, Weng PW, et al. Extracorporeal shockwave therapy improves short-term functional outcomes of shoulder adhesive capsulitis. J Shoulder Elbow Surg 2014;23(12). https://doi.org/10.1016/j.jse.2014.08.010.
58. Santoboni F, Balducci S, D'Errico V, et al. Extracorporeal shockwave therapy improves functional outcomes of adhesive capsulitis of the shoulder in patients with diabetes. Diabetes care 2017;40(2). https://doi.org/10.2337/dc16-2063.
59. Rouhani A, Mardani-Kivi M, Bazavar M, et al. Calcitonin effects on shoulder adhesive capsulitis. Eur J orthopaedic Surg Traumatol 2016;26(6). https://doi.org/10.1007/s00590-016-1816-5.
60. Kivimäki J, Pohjolainen T, Malmivaara A, et al. Manipulation under anesthesia with home exercises versus home exercises alone in the treatment of frozen shoulder: a randomized, controlled trial with 125 patients. J Shoulder Elbow Surg 2007; 16(6). https://doi.org/10.1016/j.jse.2007.02.125.
61. Melzer C, Wallny T, Wirth CJ, et al. Frozen shoulder–treatment and results. Arch Orthop Trauma Surg 1995;114(2). https://doi.org/10.1007/BF00422832.
62. Smitherman JA, Struk AM, Cricchio M, et al. Arthroscopy and manipulation versus home therapy program in treatment of adhesive capsulitis of the shoulder: a prospective randomized study. J Surg orthopaedic Adv 2015;24(1).
63. Woods DA, Loganathan K. Recurrence of frozen shoulder after manipulation under anaesthetic (MUA). Bone Joint J 2017;99-B(6). https://doi.org/10.1302/0301-620X.99B6.BJJ-2016-1133.R1.
64. Baums MH, Spahn G, Nozaki M, et al. Functional outcome and general health status in patients after arthroscopic release in adhesive capsulitis. Knee Surg Sports Traumatol Arthrosc 2007;15(5). https://doi.org/10.1007/s00167-006-0203-x.
65. Jerosch J, Nasef NM, Peters O, et al. Mid-term results following arthroscopic capsular release in patients with primary and secondary adhesive shoulder capsulitis. Knee Surg Sports Traumatol Arthrosc 2013;21(5). https://doi.org/10.1007/s00167-012-2124-1.
66. Watson L, Dalziel R, Story I. Frozen shoulder: a 12-month clinical outcome trial. J Shoulder Elbow Surg 2000;9(1). https://doi.org/10.1016/s1058-2746(00)90004-1.
67. le Lievre HMJ, Murrell GAC. Long-term outcomes after arthroscopic capsular release for idiopathic adhesive capsulitis. J bone Jt Surg Am volume 2012; 94(13). https://doi.org/10.2106/JBJS.J.00952.
68. Sivasubramanian H, Chua CXK, Lim SY, et al. Arthroscopic capsular release to treat idiopathic frozen shoulder: How much release is needed? Orthopaedics Traumatol Surg Res : OTSR 2021;107(1). https://doi.org/10.1016/j.otsr.2020.102766.
69. Miyazaki AN, Santos PD, Silva LA, et al. Avaliação dos resultados do tratamento artroscópico da capsulite adesiva do ombro. Revista Brasileira de Ortopedia 2017;52(1). https://doi.org/10.1016/j.rbo.2016.04.001.

70. Lafosse L, Boyle S, Kordasiewicz B, et al. Arthroscopic arthrolysis for recalcitrant frozen shoulder: a lateral approach. Arthroscopy 2012;28(7). https://doi.org/10.1016/j.arthro.2011.12.014.

71. Ranalletta M, Rossi LA, Zaidenberg EE, et al. Midterm outcomes after arthroscopic anteroinferior capsular release for the treatment of idiopathic adhesive capsulitis. J Arthroscopic Relat Surg 2017;33(3). https://doi.org/10.1016/j.arthro.2016.08.024.

72. Kim YS, Lee HJ, Park IJ. Clinical outcomes do not support arthroscopic posterior capsular release in addition to anterior release for shoulder stiffness. Am J Sports Med 2014;42(5). https://doi.org/10.1177/0363546514523720.

73. Ide J, Takagi K. Early and long-term results of arthroscopic treatment for shoulder stiffness. J Shoulder Elbow Surg 2004;13(2). https://doi.org/10.1016/j.jse.2003.11.001.

74. Nicholson GP. Arthroscopic capsular release for stiff shoulders. Arthrosc J Arthroscopic Relat Surg 2003;19(1). https://doi.org/10.1053/jars.2003.50010.

75. Berghs BM, Sole-Molins X, Bunker TD. Arthroscopic release of adhesive capsulitis. J Shoulder Elbow Surg 2004;13(2). https://doi.org/10.1016/j.jse.2003.12.004.

76. Boutefnouchet T, Jordan R, Bhabra G, et al. Comparison of outcomes following arthroscopic capsular release for idiopathic, diabetic and secondary shoulder adhesive capsulitis: a systematic review. Orthopaedics Traumatol Surg Res 2019;105(5). https://doi.org/10.1016/j.otsr.2019.02.014.

77. Jerosch J, Filler TJ, Peuker ET. Which joint position puts the axillary nerve at lowest risk when performing arthroscopic capsular release in patients with adhesive capsulitis of the shoulder? Knee Surg Sports Traumatol Arthrosc : official J ESSKA 2002;10(2). https://doi.org/10.1007/s00167-001-0270-y.

78. Berndt T, Elki S, Sedlinsch A, et al. Arthroskopische arthrolyse bei schultersteife. Oper Orthopädie Traumatologie 2015;27(2). https://doi.org/10.1007/s00064-013-0284-x.

79. Nunez FA, Papadonikolakis A, Li Z. Arthroscopic release of adhesive capsulitis of the shoulder complicated with shoulder dislocation and brachial plexus injury. J Surg orthopaedic Adv 2016;25(2).

Postoperative Rehabilitation After Shoulder Arthroplasty

William Polio, MD, Tyler J. Brolin, MD*

KEYWORDS

- Total shoulder arthroplasty • Anatomic total shoulder arthroplasty
- Reverse total shoulder arthroplasty • Physical therapy protocol
- Postoperative rehabilitation

KEY POINTS

- Postoperative rehabilitation is standard practice after total shoulder arthroplasty (TSA), and reliably good outcomes have been obtained despite considerable diversity in rehabilitation programs, with home-based physical therapy (PT) being at least as effective as supervised PT.
- After anatomic TSA (aTSA), the greatest gains in forward flexion and external rotation (ER) strength occur between 3 and 6 months, and patients continue to see strength improvement up to 1 year.
- After reverse TSA (rTSA), the greatest gains in forward flexion strength occur from 0 to 3 months and ER strength from 6 months to 1 year. Strength improvement in forward flexion can be seen for up to 1 year and in ER for up to 2 years. Internal rotation motion can improve for up to 2 years.
- After rTSA, outcomes after accelerated rehabilitation are noninferior and may benefit the elderly by reducing fall risk and allowing them to return to activities of daily living sooner.

INTRODUCTION

Total shoulder arthroplasty (TSA), including anatomic (aTSA) and reverse total shoulder arthroplasty (rTSA), is an increasingly popular operation due to its ability to achieve reliably good clinical outcomes through decreasing pain and improving function. aTSA is indicated for end-stage glenohumeral degenerative conditions in patients with sufficient rotator cuff and glenohumeral bone stock.[1] Unlike aTSA, rTSA indications have expanded into a broad category encompassing glenohumeral degenerative conditions with insufficient rotator cuff and/or bone stock, which include end-stage cuff

University of Tennessee Health Science Center-Campbell Clinic, 1211 Union Avenue, Suite 510, Memphis, TN 38104, USA
* Corresponding author.
E-mail address: tbrolin@campbellclinic.com

Phys Med Rehabil Clin N Am 34 (2023) 469–479
https://doi.org/10.1016/j.pmr.2022.12.010
1047-9651/23/© 2022 Elsevier Inc. All rights reserved.

pmr.theclinics.com

tear arthropathy, massive irreparable rotator cuff tears, inflammatory and noninflammatory arthritis, proximal humerus fractures, failed hemiarthroplasty or aTSA, and tumors of the proximal humerus, all of which, contribute to the overall increased incidence of shoulder arthroplasty. Similar to hip and knee arthroplasty, postoperative physical therapy (PT) is considered essential to the success of the operation and has become standard practice. However, there is a paucity of high-quality research evaluating PT programs after TSA, which has led to significant diversity in postoperative rehabilitation programs. There is no clear consensus regarding when to initiate passive, active-assisted, and resistance exercises, the tolerance limits of shoulder range of motion (ROM) at specific time points, the value of formal PT compared with a home exercise program, and short- and long-term precautions.[2]

Neer[3] originally described the principles in shoulder rehabilitation that are still used today, which include early ROM in a protected and graduated manner to minimize scar formation and muscle atrophy and protect healing tissue.[3] Typically, rehabilitation programs are designed to regain active elevation by starting with gravity-minimized exercises and progressing to inclined and upright assisted elevation exercises.[4] For aTSA, subscapularis protection is the most important restraint of the postoperative rehabilitation program. Passive and active tension on the tendon should be limited by restricting external rotation (ER), passive ROM (PROM), and active internal rotation (IR) exercises.[2] In rTSA, subscapularis integrity is not as critical for successful outcomes and restraints in rehabilitation protocols are aimed more toward preventing dislocations and acromial stress fractures.[1] In addition, rehabilitation protocols after rTSA must account for the alteration in moment arms of the shoulder girdle musculature due to its nonanatomic design.[5] The purpose of this review was to describe the current principles and controversies of rehabilitation after TSA.

GENERAL REHABILITATION PRINCIPLES

Most postoperative rehabilitation protocols after TSA are based on expert opinion informed by biomechanical principles. Few randomized control trials exist to guide the development of a rehabilitation program. However, some common elements are found across most studies. Typically, protocols divide the rehabilitation pathway into three or four sequential phases with suggestive timeframes and functional goals. The initial postoperative recovery phase lasts from 2 to 6 weeks and is focused on wound healing, edema control, pain management, and a gradual introduction of PROM exercises. In the case of aTSA, maximal protection of the subscapularis repair limits ER in this phase, whereas in rTSA a position of adduction, extension, and IR is avoided to prevent dislocation. The next phase, typically between 6 and 12 weeks postoperatively, begins active ROM (AROM) exercises and progressive strengthening beginning with isometric exercises. The final phase begins at 12 weeks postoperatively and can last up to a year and involves functional strengthening exercises and transition to a home exercise program.[1]

Progression from gentle PROM to AROM that ultimately incorporates strengthening must balance being too protective, which can result in stiffness, and being too aggressive, which could jeopardize the integrity of subscapularis repair or prosthesis stability.[6] Biomechanical data suggest that active assisted ROM (AAROM) exercises produce muscular demand levels that are intermediate between PROM and AROM exercises, making them useful to bridge the gap in rehabilitation programs between PROM and AROM. AAROM exercises can be further subdivided into gravity-minimized and upright-assistive exercises. Gravity-minimized elevation exercises for the anterior deltoid have been shown to result in a low relative muscle demand, similar to PROM exercises. Upright-assistive elevation exercises have been shown to result in low to moderate relative muscle demand, in contrast to an active elevation that is moderate demand. This suggests that a rehabilitation program progressing from PROM to gravity minimized to upright assistive to AROM exercises would minimize large jumps in muscular demands while restoring AROM.[4]

Poor preoperative ROM and function have been shown to negatively affect postoperative ROM and outcomes after TSA.[7] This may be the result of chronic deltoid deconditioning and/or rotator cuff dysfunction, in addition to cortical adaptations in the brain.[8] In a study of rTSA, a poor Constant Score in the contralateral, nonoperative arm also was predictive of poorer ROM recovery in the operative arm. This indicates that self-directed rehabilitation protocols using the contralateral arm to perform active assist functions may be beneficial compared with those more heavily reliant on physical therapist assistance.[9]

TSA results in sustained predictable improvements in pain scores, functional scores, and ROM.[10–12] The rate of recovery after surgery has been investigated for both aTSA and rTSA. Patients undergoing rTSA were older with worse preoperative functional scores and ROM, which affected the speed of recovery after surgery. The plateau in maximal recovery was quicker and more predictable for patients undergoing aTSA. At 6 months, 90% to 100% of functional improvement had been achieved in patients undergoing aTSA versus 72% to 90% of functional improvement in rTSA. Improvements in ROM were 80% to 92% for both aTSA and rTSA at 6 months, with the exception of IR improvement in rTSA. Pain scores improved more rapidly, with 85% improvement at 3 months in both aTSA and rTSA. Patients undergoing aTSA reached plateaus for improvements in pain scores, functional scores and abduction at 6 months and forward flexion and IR at 1 year and ER at 2 years. The plateau in improvement for patients undergoing rTSA was more variable, with slow and sustained improvements over 2 years.[13]

REHABILITATION AFTER ANATOMIC TOTAL SHOULDER ARTHROPLASTY

Successful subscapularis repair is critical to the outcome of aTSA. Subscapularis failure is associated with anterior shoulder instability, pain, lower patient-reported outcomes, and weakness in shoulder IR. Regardless of subscapularis takedown and repair technique, the clinically significant subscapularis re-tear rate is around 3%.[2] Postoperative rehabilitation after aTSA is a balance between protection of the subscapular repair and joint mobilization. No consensus exists on duration and type of sling immobilization, with protocols existing ranging from 24 h to 6 weeks of sling use.[14] In a randomized control trial, Baumgarten and colleagues[15] evaluated the influence of arm position during sling use after aTSA. Significantly greater improvements in ROM changes from baseline to final follow-up were found in the group using a neutral rotation sling compared with an IR sling for active ER (42 vs 25°), passive ER (44 vs 26°), and passive horizontal adduction (7.7 cm vs 3.7 cm), along with a trend toward improved active IR behind the back (18 cm vs 11 cm, $P = .09$). In addition, the neutral sling group had significantly less night pain at 2 weeks.[15]

Stiffness is a common complaint in patients who are unsatisfied after aTSA.[16] Early PROM traditionally has been advocated to avoid postoperative stiffness; however, there is no consensus on specific parameters or limitations. In general, passive shoulder ER and active IR should be limited to protect the subscapularis repair. Most studies describe restricting passive ER to 30 to 40° for a period of time postoperatively, whereas some restrict ER to neutral. Forward flexion restrictions have been described from 90° to 130° to unrestricted in the immediate postoperative period.[14]

Cadaveric studies suggest that passive shoulder elevation is safe after subscapularis repair,[17] but restriction to ER and abduction may be beneficial to healing.[18,19]

There is one randomized control trial to suggest that initiation of early ROM exercises after aTSA promotes significantly quicker return of function and improvement in pain in the short term (4 to 8 weeks) that is not upheld at 3 months or beyond. Denard and colleagues[20] compared ROM and outcome scores between patients treated with either an immediate or delayed motion protocol after aTSA with a lesser tuberosity osteotomy. Both groups used a sling for 4 weeks. The immediate motion group began unlimited passive forward flexion exercises and ER to 30° on postoperative day (POD) 1, along with active elbow, wrist, and hand exercises and active scapular retraction. At 4 weeks, the sling was discontinued, and active forward flexion and unlimited passive ER exercises were permitted. At 8 weeks strengthening was initiated and patients were released to activities as tolerated at 12 weeks. The delayed motion group began active hand, wrist, and elbow exercises on POD 1 along with scapular retraction exercises but delayed passive forward flexion and ER until 4 weeks when the sling was discontinued. At 8 weeks, AROM was allowed, and strengthening was initiated. Patients were released to activities as tolerated at 16 weeks. At 4 weeks the immediate motion group had better improvement in function than the delayed group as measured by the ASES score and at 8 weeks as measured by the American Shoulder and Elbow Surgeons (ASES) and Single Assessment Numeric Evaluation (SANE) scores. Also at 8 weeks, the immediate motion group had better improvement in the visual analog scale (VAS) score. At all other time points, including 1 year, the groups did not differ in outcome scores. At no time point did the group differ in ROM in any plane. No significant difference was found in lesser tuberosity healing rates; however, a trend was apparent toward lower healing rate in the immediate motion group compared with the delayed motion (82% vs 96%, $P = .10$). Although not statistically significant, it is important clinically because patients without radiographic lesser tuberosity osteotomy healing had lower ASES scores, which is consistent with existing literature.[20,21]

Differences in subscapularis management during exposure and closure complicate comparisons of rehabilitation protocols after aTSA; however, there may be little clinical or functional downside to delaying PROM. The benefit of formal PT compared with a home exercise program after aTSA has also been challenged. In a level III retrospective review, Mulieri and colleagues[6] investigated the difference in outcomes between a group of patients treated with immediate motion in PT and those treated with delayed motion for 6 weeks and a physician-directed home exercise program after aTSA. Both groups underwent a subscapularis tenotomy and used a shoulder immobilizer for 6 weeks. The PT group was allowed passive elevation in the scapular plane to 120° and ER to 20° during the first 3 weeks postoperatively under the direction of a physical therapist. Supine AAROM and isometric shoulder exercises were begun at 4 weeks, AROM at 7 weeks, and strengthening exercises at 10 weeks. The home program groups were allowed pendulum exercises the first 6 to 8 weeks until the shoulder immobilizer was discontinued. At that time, they began supine AAROM forward flexion exercises and were allowed to use their arm for activities of daily living (ADLs). After 14 weeks, patients were released to activities as tolerated. No differences were found at any time point for ASES or Subjective Shoulder Test (SST) scores. At 3 months, a significant difference in IR was found (PT group L1, home program group L5, $P \le .002$); however, this difference was not sustained at any other time point. There was no difference in forward flexion and abduction at 3, 6, or 12 months; however, at the final follow-up (PT 52 months vs Home 39 months) forward flexion (119° vs 154°) and abduction (108° vs 147°) were significantly better in the home program group.[6]

Improvement in shoulder activity levels after aTSA is associated with improvements in strength. Baumgarten and colleagues[22] showed that strength improvements compared with the preoperative state are associated with greater improvements in outcome scores and ROM.[22] As scapulothoracic motion contributes more to overall shoulder ROM after TSA than in the native shoulder,[23] periscapular muscle strengthening is often initiated early in the rehabilitation course with retraction and protraction exercises. This is important for reestablishing neuromuscular scapular control and minimizes stress across the glenohumeral joint. After subscapularis healing, rotator cuff strengthening is started to maximize glenohumeral motion and stability.[14] After aTSA, patients continue to see strength improvements in forward flexion and ER up to 1 year. The greatest gains in forward flexion and ER strength occur between 3 and 6 months.[24]

The authors preferred rehabilitation protocol is shown below. Patients undergo a one-time PT visit at the 2 weeks postoperatively to learn a home rehabilitation program. Formal PT is initiated for twice per week beginning at 6 weeks. At 12 weeks, patients begin transitioning to a home rehabilitation program based on the progress of their rehabilitation.

ANATOMIC TOTAL SHOULDER ARTHROPLASTY REHABILITATION PROTOCOL

- 0 to 2 weeks: Phase 1 stretching
  - Codman exercises
  - Assisted forward elevation to 90°
  - Assisted ER to neutral degrees
- 2 to 6 weeks: Phase 2 stretching
  - Phase 2 stretching initiated (limit FE to 140°, ER to 40°)
    - Continue previous exercises
    - Assisted elevation with pulleys
    - Assisted abduction
- 6 to 12 weeks: Phase 3 stretching, Phase 1 strengthening
  - Phase 3 stretching initiated (no limits)
    - Continue previous exercises
    - Assisted FE and ER stretches using the doorway
    - Assisted IR
    - Assisted adduction
  - Phase 1 Strengthening initiated
    - Isometric forward elevation, extension, and ER with arm in neutral
    - Supine active forward elevation (beginning with the elbow flexed and controlled decline progressing up to 5 lbs)
- Greater than 12 weeks: Phase 2 strengthening
  - Phase 2 strengthening initiated
    - Seated active forward elevation
    - Theraband exercises working on anterior, middle, and posterior deltoid, and IR/ER
    - Progress to home exercise program

REHABILITATION AFTER REVERSE TOTAL SHOULDER ARTHROPLASTY

Rehabilitation after rTSA must be considered separately from aTSA for several reasons. rTSA is a nonanatomic reconstruction that relies on changes in joint biomechanics due to alteration of muscle moment arms and length-tension relationships to achieve restoration of motion that is not reliant on the rotator cuff. Healing of the subscapularis is not as critical for outcomes and early rehabilitation precautions are more focused on prevention of instability and acromial/scapular spine stress fractures.[25] Avoidance of exercises that result in combined shoulder extension, adduction, and IR (hand behind the back posture) in early postoperative rehabilitation period is thought to mitigate the risk of prosthetic instability.[2] Most dislocations occur within the first 6 weeks after rTSA, with few occurring after 3 months. Since early instability is more of a concern in rTSA than aTSA, a higher level of consensus exists for sling utilization during the first 4 to 6 weeks postoperatively.[14]

rTSA moves the joint center of rotation medial and inferior that increases the moment arm of the deltoid to recruit more fibers during elevation. In contrast to the native shoulder, in which the anterior deltoid is mainly a flexor, middle deltoid is mainly an abductor, and posterior deltoid is mainly an extensor, all three heads contribute to abduction after rTSA. The most effective flexors after rTSA are the anterior deltoid and superior pectoralis major, with lesser contribution from the middle deltoid.[5] Increased preoperative deltoid size has been shown to positively correlate with improved postoperative Constant and ASES scores, as well as SST and strength; whereas increased preoperative fatty infiltration of the deltoid has been shown to be associated with lower postoperative ASES scores.[26] Although many rehabilitation protocols acknowledge the importance of deltoid strengthening after rTSA, there is no consensus on when to initiate strengthening exercises, which must balance concerns of acromial stress fracture and implant loosening.[27] In contrast to aTSA, the greatest gains in forward flexion strength occur from 0 to 3 months postoperatively for rTSA. Strength improvement in forward flexion can be seen for up to 1 year.[24] Return of functional ER after rTSA is less predictable than forward flexion. Electrophysiological data suggest that active ER beyond neutral in rTSA is powered equally and sequentially by the teres minor, teres major, and posterior deltoid. Strengthening protocols should attempt to incorporate these muscles to maximize ER.[28] In contrast to aTSA, the greatest gain in ER strength after rTSA occurs between 6 months and 1 year, with improvement being seen for up to 2 years.[24]

Controversy exists regarding the necessity of subscapularis repair during rTSA. In medialized prosthetic designs, repair of the subscapularis is associated with increased prosthetic stability[29]; however, in lateralized prosthetic designs, repair of the subscapularis has not been shown to impart increased stability.[30] In addition, an intact subscapularis may provide improved shoulder IR, which is a critical motion for self-care.[31] Triplet and colleagues[32] found that although 67% of patients after aTSA achieved IR to T12, only 32% of patients after rTSA were able to achieve this level of IR. Some authors have suggested a more aggressive rehabilitation program after rTSA due to less reliance on subscapularis function, particularly in lateralized rTSA designs; however, if repaired, consideration can be given to subscapularis protection during the early phases of rehabilitation. IR ROM after rTSA can be expected to improve up to 2 years.[9]

There is no consensus regarding the initiation and limitations of PROM or AROM after rTSA. The main concerns relate to prosthetic instability, acromial stress fracture, and, if repaired, subscapularis healing. Edwards and colleagues[27] conducted a randomized control trial to determine if early deltoid and active rotator exercises (EA) compared with delayed active, deltoid-only exercises (DA) would result in significantly improved shoulder strength and ROM after rTSA. Patients were immobilized with a sling for 6 weeks and underwent the same rehabilitation for the first 2 weeks after surgery. In the DA group, a home-based program was initiated at 2 weeks that incorporated PROM exercises until 6 weeks, followed by AAROM exercises from 6 to 12 weeks. At 12 weeks, patients returned to activities as tolerated with no additional formal rehabilitation. In the EA group, a home-based program was initiated at 2 weeks that incorporated PROM and select AAROM exercises, as well as isometric deltoid strengthening until 6 weeks. From 6 to 12 weeks, graduated AAROM and AROM exercises were initiated, along with ER strengthening exercises. After 12 weeks, formal PT was prescribed for strengthening of the deltoid, internal and external rotators, and scapulothoracic muscles. No differences were found between the groups in terms of complication rate, ROM, functional outcome (ASES, Global Shoulder Function [GSF], SANE) or pain (VAS) scores, with the exception of improved forward flexion in the EA ROM group at 3 months and more patients in the EA group obtaining the MCID in the GSF from 3 to 6 months (76% vs 43%, $P = .016$). This led the authors to conclude that early, active rehabilitation is safe and effective and may have early benefits over a delayed rehabilitation program.[27]

Hagen and colleagues[33] conducted a randomized control trial comparing a group of patients with immobilization and no PROM or AROM for 6 weeks with a group of patients allowed immediate PROM and AROM (with forward flexion strengthening delayed until 6 weeks and ER strengthening delayed until 12 weeks). They found no difference in terms of complication rates, outcome scores, or ROM with the exception of improved ASES pain scores at 6 months in the delayed rehabilitation group. This led the authors to suggest that early ROM protocols are safe and may benefit the elderly population by avoiding the limitations of prolonged immobilization.[33] Lee and colleagues[34] compared the outcomes of patients treated an accelerated rehabilitation protocol and no immobilization with those treated with more a conservative rehabilitation program and either 6 or 3 weeks of sling immobilization. The patients were allocated to each rehabilitation group chronologically, as the senior surgeons postoperative rehabilitation program evolved overtime. The earliest group underwent 6 weeks of sling immobilization and immediate initiation of PROM, with initiation of AAROM at 3 weeks and AROM and resisted deltoid rehabilitation at 6 weeks. The next group underwent 3 weeks of sling immobilization and immediate initiation of PROM and AAROM, with initiation of AROM and resisted deltoid rehabilitation at 3 weeks. In the accelerated rehabilitation group, patients were placed in a sling only as long as the interscalene block was in place (1 to 2 days) and allowed to progress immediately from PROM to AAROM to AROM and anterior deltoid strengthening regime as pain tolerated. These patients were allowed to use their arm as tolerated for all their regular activity with the exception of forced or weight-bearing combined shoulder adduction, extension, and IR. No differences between groups were found at 3 weeks, 3 months, 6 months, 9 months, or 1 year in terms of Constant score, SSV, VAS, ROM, or return to work, sport, or leisure activity. A higher number of complications were found in the 6 weeks immobilization group than in the 3 week or accelerated rehabilitation group, mostly related to periprosthetic fracture from falls (17 vs 3 vs 3). This led the authors to conclude that outcomes after accelerated rehabilitation are noninferior and may be particularly beneficial to the elderly because of improved proprioception and balance when not wearing a sling and the ability to return to daily life activities immediately.[34]

The authors' preferred rehabilitation protocol is shown below. Patients undergo a one-time PT visit at the 2 weeks postoperatively to learn a home rehabilitation program. Formal PT is initiated for twice per week beginning at 6 weeks. At 12 weeks, patients begin transitioning to a home rehabilitation program based on the progress of their rehabilitation.

Reverse Total Shoulder Arthroplasty Rehabilitation Protocol

- 0 to 2 weeks: Phase 1 stretching

- Pendulum exercises
- Assisted forward elevation to 90°
- Assisted ER to 30°
- Hand, wrist, elbow ROM
- Edema control
- 2 to 6 weeks: Phase 2 stretching, Phase 1 strengthening
  - Sling discontinued throughout day at 2 weeks. Patients to wear sling while sleeping until 6 weeks postoperatively.
  - Restriction include nonweight-bearing on affected extremity, avoidance of pushing off with affected extremity while rising from seated position, no IR behind the back, no lifting with affected extremity.
  - **Single PT visit at 2 weeks to educate on Phase 2 stretching and Phase 1 strengthening exercises.**
  - Phase 2 stretching initiated (limit FE to 140°, ER to 40°)
    - Continue previous stretching exercises
    - Assisted elevation with pulleys
    - Assisted abduction
  - Phase 1 strengthening
    - Initiate deltoid strengthening exercises by beginning in supine position with arm flexed and progressing to seated position using body weight only.
- 6 to 12 weeks: Phase 3 stretching, Phase 2 strengthening
  - Phase 3 stretching initiated (no limits)
    - Continue previous exercises
    - Assisted FE and ER stretches using doorway
    - Assisted IR
    - Assisted adduction
  - Phase 2 strengthening initiated
    - Isometric forward elevation, extension, and ER with arm in neutral
    - Continue deltoid strengthening up to 5-lb weights in supine position and progressing to 5-lb weights in seated position
- >12 weeks: Phase 3 strengthening
  - Phase 3 strengthening initiated
    - Theraband exercises working on anterior, middle, and posterior deltoid as well as IR/ER
    - Progress to home exercise program

SUMMARY

Although TSA has become an increasingly popular operation due to reliably good outcomes, there still exists significant diversity in postoperative rehabilitation programs. Different concerns exist in the early postoperative period after aTSA and rTSA, which has led to variations in postoperative rehabilitation programs between these two procedures. In addition to variations in postoperative rehabilitation, there is no consensus on long-term limitations after TSA. Traditionally, activities such as overhead sports, weight-lifting, and heavy manual labor were restricted after TSA, and patients were given a 20-lb lifting restriction. However, these limitations were set at the surgeon's discretion, with little support in evidence-based literature.[35] Recent studies suggest that patients have a strong predilection to return to activities they participated in before surgery. Patients returned to sports at a rate of 93% after aTSA and 75% after rTSA. The most common sports patients participated in were swimming, golf, and tennis.[36] The only long-term restriction given to patients by the authors are to avoid repetitive overhead lifting greater than 20 lbs.

An estimated 70,000 TSA are performed each year in the United States alone.[1] As the burden of health care costs continues to rise, the benefit of formal PT after TSA must be weighed against its cost. Cost not only includes the price of each PT session, but lost time and cost of travel to and from therapy for the patients and, when necessary, caregiver, which is common considering the number of elderly patients undergoing TSA.[27] Home-based exercise programs have been shown to be effective after both aTSA and rTSA; however, patients may benefit in the early postoperative period with more accelerated rehabilitation programs that often require guidance from a physical therapist.[6,27] In patients returning to work, hoping to resume an active lifestyle more quickly, or who are slowly progressing after surgery, the benefits of formal PT likely outweigh the increased cost.

CLINICS CARE POINTS

- Postoperative rehabilitation is standard practice after total shoulder arthroplasty (TSA), and reliably good outcomes have been obtained despite considerable diversity in rehabilitation programs.

- Poor preoperative range of motion (ROM) and function have been shown to predict poorer postoperative ROM and outcomes after TSA

- After anatomic TSA (aTSA), the greatest gains in forward flexion and external rotation (ER) strength occur between 3 and 6 months and patients continue to see strength improvements up to 1 year.

- After reverse TSA (rTSA), the greatest gains in forward flexion strength occur from 0 to 3 months and ER strength from 6 months to 1 year. Strength improvement in forward flexion can be seen for up to 1 year and in ER up to 2 years. Internal rotation (IR) motion can improve for up to 2 years.

- For aTSA, subscapularis protection is the most important restraint of the postoperative rehabilition program, whereas for rTSA subscapularis integrity is not as critical for successful outcomes and restraints are aimed more toward preventing dislocations and acromial stress fractures

- One randomized control trial showed significantly greater improvements in ROM in patients using a neutral rotation sling compared with an IR sling after aTSA

- One randomized control trial suggested that initiation of early ROM exercises after aTSA promotes the significantly quicker return of function and improvement in pain in the short term (4 to 8 weeks) but not 3 months or beyond. A nonstatistically significant trend was found toward lower lesser tuberosity osteotomy healing rates in the accelerated rehabilitation group.

- After rTSA, outcomes after accelerated rehabilitation are noninferior and may benefit the elderly by reducing fall risk and allowing them to return to activities of daily living sooner.

DISCLOSURE

Dr T.J. Brolin reports board or committee memberships with American Shoulder and Elbow Surgeons and Orthopedic Clinics of North America and financial relationships with Arthrex, Inc., DJ Orthopedics, Elsevier, and Orthofix, Inc. The authors report no conflicts of interest.

REFERENCES

1. Bullock GS, Garrigues GE, Ledbetter L, et al. A systematic review of proposed rehabilitation guidelines following anatomic and reverse shoulder arthroplasty. J Orthop Sports Phys Ther 2019;49(5):337–46.
2. Levy DM, Abrams GD, Harris JD, et al. Rotator cuff tears after total shoulder arthroplasty in primary osteoarthritis: a systematic review. Int J Shoulder Surg 2016; 10(2):78–84.
3. Hughes M, Neer CS 2nd. Glenohumeral joint replacement and postoperative rehabilitation. Phys Ther 1975;55(8):850–8.
4. Gaunt BW, McCluskey GM, Uhl TL. An electromyographic evaluation of subdividing active-assistive shoulder elevation exercises. Sports Health 2010;2(5): 424–32.
5. Ackland DC, Roshan-Zamir S, Richardson M, et al. Moment arms of the shoulder musculature after reverse total shoulder arthroplasty. J Bone Joint Surg Am 2010; 92(5):1221–30.
6. Mulieri PJ, Holcomb JO, Dunning P, et al. Is a formal physical therapy program necessary after total shoulder arthroplasty for osteoarthritis? J Shoulder Elbow Surg 2010;19(4):570–9.
7. Friedman RJ, Eichinger J, Schoch B, et al. Preoperative parameters that predict postoperative patient-reported outcome measures and range of motion with anatomic and reverse total shoulder arthroplasty. JSES Open Access 2019; 3(4):266–72.
8. Haller S, Cunningham G, Laedermann A, et al. Shoulder apprehension impacts large-scale functional brain networks. AJNR Am J Neuroradiol 2014;35(4):691–7.
9. Collin P, Matsukawa T, Denard PJ, et al. Pre-operative factors influence the recovery of range of motion following reverse shoulder arthroplasty. Int Orthop 2017; 41(10):2135–42.
10. Boileau P, Watkinson D, Hatzidakis AM, et al. Neer Award 2005: The Grammont reverse shoulder prosthesis: results in cuff tear arthritis, fracture sequelae, and revision arthroplasty. J Shoulder Elbow Surg 2006;15(5):527–40.
11. Deshmukh AV, Koris M, Zurakowski D, et al. Total shoulder arthroplasty: long-term survivorship, functional outcome, and quality of life. J Shoulder Elbow Surg 2005; 14(5):471–9.
12. Norris TR, Iannotti JP. Functional outcome after shoulder arthroplasty for primary osteoarthritis: a multicenter study. J Shoulder Elbow Surg 2002;11(2):130–5.
13. Levy JC, Everding NG, Gil CC Jr, et al. Speed of recovery after shoulder arthroplasty: a comparison of reverse and anatomic total shoulder arthroplasty. J Shoulder Elbow Surg 2014;23(12):1872–81.
14. Kirsch JM, Namdari S. Rehabilitation after anatomic and reverse total shoulder arthroplasty: a critical analysis review. JBJS Rev 2020;8(2):e0129.
15. Baumgarten KM, Osborn R, Schweinle WE 3rd, et al. The position of sling immobilization influences the outcomes of anatomic total shoulder arthroplasty: a randomized, single-blind, prospective study. J Shoulder Elbow Surg 2018;27(12): 2120–8.
16. Hasan SS, Leith JM, Campbell B, et al. Characteristics of unsatisfactory shoulder arthroplasties. J Shoulder Elbow Surg 2002;11(5):431–41.
17. Uhl TL, Muir TA, Lawson L. Electromyographical assessment of passive, active assistive, and active shoulder rehabilitation exercises. PM R 2010;2(2):132–41.
18. Muraki T, Aoki M, Uchiyama E, et al. A cadaveric study of strain on the subscapularis muscle. Arch Phys Med Rehabil 2007;88(7):941–6.

19. Wright T, Easley T, Bennett J, et al. Shoulder arthroplasty and its effect on strain in the subscapularis muscle. Clin Biomech (Bristol, Avon) 2015;30(4):373–6.
20. Denard PJ, Ladermann A. Immediate versus delayed passive range of motion following total shoulder arthroplasty. J Shoulder Elbow Surg 2016;25:1918–24.
21. Jackson JD, Cil A, Smith J, et al. Integrity and function of the subscapularis after total shoulder arthroplasty. J Shoulder Elbow Surg 2010;19(7):1085–90.
22. Baumgarten KM, Osborn R, Schweinle WE Jr, et al. The influence of anatomic total shoulder arthroplasty using a subscapularis tenotomy on shoulder strength. J Shoulder Elbow Surg 2018;27(1):82–9.
23. de Toledo JM, Loss JF, Janssen TW, et al. Kinematic evaluation of patients with total and reverse shoulder arthroplasty during rehabilitation exercises with different loads. Clin Biomech (Bristol, Avon) 2012;27(8):793–800.
24. Hao KA, Wright TW, Schoch BS, et al. Rate of improvement in shoulder strength after anatomic and reverse total shoulder arthroplasty. JSES Int 2021;6(2):247–52.
25. Edwards PK, Ebert JR, Littlewood C, et al. Effectiveness of formal physical therapy following total shoulder arthroplasty: A systematic review. Shoulder Elbow 2020;12(2):136–43.
26. Wiater BP, Koueiter DM, Maerz T, et al. Preoperative deltoid size and fatty infiltration of the deltoid and rotator cuff correlate to outcomes after reverse total shoulder arthroplasty. Clin Orthop Relat Res 2015;473(2):663–73.
27. Edwards PK, Ebert JR, Joss B, et al. A randomised trial comparing two rehabilitation approaches following reverse total shoulder arthroplasty. Shoulder Elbow 2021;13(5):557–72.
28. Polio W, Hajek B, Brolin TJ, et al. Muscle activation patterns during aER after RTSA: an electrophysiological study of the teres minor and associated musculature. Poster presented at: San Diego Shoulder Institute 39th annual Shoulder Course; 2022 June 15–18; Coronado, CA.
29. Edwards TB, Williams MD, Labriola JE, et al. Subscapularis insufficiency and the risk of shoulder dislocation after reverse shoulder arthroplasty. J Shoulder Elbow Surg 2009;18(6):892–6.
30. Roberson TA, Shanley E, Griscom JT, et al. Subscapularis repair Is unnecessary after lateralized reverse shoulder arthroplasty. JB JS Open Access 2018;3(3):e0056.
31. Dedy NJ, Gouk CJ, Taylor FJ, et al. Sonographic assessment of the subscapularis after reverse shoulder arthroplasty: impact of tendon integrity on shoulder function. J Shoulder Elbow Surg 2018;27:1051–6.
32. Triplet JJ, Everding NG, Levy JC, et al. Functional internal rotation after shoulder arthroplasty: a comparison of anatomic and reverse shoulder arthroplasty. J Shoulder Elbow Surg 2015;24:867–74.
33. Hagen MS, Allahabadi S, Zhang AL, et al. A randomized single-blinded trial of early rehabilitation versus immobilization after reverse total shoulder arthroplasty. J Shoulder Elbow Surg 2020;29(3):442–50.
34. Lee J, Consigliere P, Fawzy E, et al. Accelerated rehabilitation following reverse total shoulder arthroplasty. J Shoulder Elbow Surg 2021;30(9):e545–57.
35. Romeo AA. Activity limitations after shoulder arthroplasty: Be all you can be. Orthopaedic Proc 2019;101-B(No. SUPP 8).
36. Liu JN, Steinhaus ME, Garcia GH, et al. Return to sport after shoulder arthroplasty: a systematic review and meta-analysis. Knee Surg Sports Traumatol Arthrosc 2018;26(1):100–12.

Muscular Retraining and Rehabilitation after Shoulder Muscle Tendon Transfer

Abdulaziz F. Ahmed, MD, Ryan Lohre, MD,
Bassem T. Elhassan, MD*

KEYWORDS

• Tendon • Transfers • Rehabilitation • Shoulder • Retraining

KEY POINTS

- Rehabilitation after shoulder muscle tendon transfers requires extensive and lengthy rehabilitation of approximately 6 months.
- Rehabilitation must consider the patient preoperative function and the severity of muscular deficits to manage patients' expectations.
- Different shoulder tendon transfers have different immobilization requirements and specific restrictions to ensure optimal soft tissue healing and functional improvement.
- The final phase of rehabilitation should be individualized to optimize the patients' return to desired activities and occupation.

INTRODUCTION

Muscle tendon transfers around the shoulder involve transferring the tendon of a well-functioning muscle–tendon unit to the site of damaged muscle–tendon insertion. In turn, this restores function and strength of the injured shoulder muscle through dynamic muscular contraction and a tenodesis effect. The most common indication for muscle tendon transfers in the shoulder are massive irreparable rotator cuff tears, especially in active and relatively younger individuals, due to the high probability of treatment failure associated with rotator cuff repair. Moreover, muscle tendon transfers are also performed for deltoid muscle deficiency, which is most performed concomitantly with a reverse shoulder arthroplasty. After shoulder tendon transfer surgery, immobilization and rehabilitation of the transferred muscle tendon are crucial to optimize clinical outcomes. In this article, we will discuss in detail the rehabilitation after muscle tendon transfer procedures.

Department of Orthopedic Surgery, Massachusetts General Hospital, Harvard Medical School, Boston, MA, USA
* Corresponding author. MGH Shoulder Service, Harvard Medical School, 55 Fruit Street, Boston MA 02114.
E-mail address: belhassan@mgh.harvard.edu

Phys Med Rehabil Clin N Am 34 (2023) 481–488
https://doi.org/10.1016/j.pmr.2023.01.001
1047-9651/23/© 2023 Elsevier Inc. All rights reserved.
pmr.theclinics.com

Muscle–Tendon Adaptation After Muscle Tendon Transfers

Several basic science studies have demonstrated cellular adaptations within skeletal muscles after altering the muscle length through joint immobilization or retinacular releases. Williams and colleagues[1] has demonstrated in mice models that immobilization of the soleus muscle in a lengthening position induced increased sarcomere production after 4 weeks of immobilization. Koh and Herzog[2] have reported similar adaptation after tibialis anterior muscle retinacular releases in rabbit models. When compared with controls, the tibialis anterior muscle tendons with retinacular release had increased excursion and moment arms similar to that in tendon transfers. Furthermore, the muscles exhibited increased sarcomeres 12-week after retinacular releases. However, Takahashi and colleagues[3] have found that this adaptation was asynchronous between a muscle and its respective tendon after tendon transfer procedures. In their study on 37 rabbit models, the extensor digitorum muscle of the second toe was transferred at a lengthened position. The authors found a significant increase in sarcomere numbers in the transferred muscle after 1 week of surgery. However, the tendon adaptation was delayed and resulted in an undesirable tendon lengthening by an average of 1.43 mm during 8 weeks after tendon transfer. These aforementioned studies provide insights on important muscle tendon adaptations that are relevant to rehabilitation after tendon transfers. However, further clinical and basic science studies are warranted to further elucidate the complex adaptation following tendon transfers.

Overview of Muscle Tendon Transfers Procedures

Muscle tendon transfers for posterosuperior cuff deficiency

Posterosuperior rotator cuff muscles include the supraspinatus, infraspinatus, and the teres minor. The main function of the supraspinatus is to initiate shoulder elevation, whereas the infraspinatus and teres minor are power external rotators of the shoulder. The main purpose of muscle tendon transfers for posterosuperior cuff deficiency is to restore shoulder external rotation and to a lesser extent to improve shoulder elevation. Deficiency of the posterosuperior cuff is treated with either the latissimus dorsi tendon transfer (with or without teres major), or the lower trapezius tendon transfer.

The latissimus dorsi muscle originates from the sacrum, T7-L5 spinous processes, and the 10th to 12th rib. Thereafter, it inserts on the proximal humerus just medial the bicipital groove and underneath the pectoralis major tendon. The latissimus dorsi tendon is a shoulder internal rotator. Thus, to achieve external rotation of the shoulder with a latissimus tendon transfer, the tendon has to wrapped posterior around the humerus, and it is then anchored onto the greater tuberosity or proximal humerus. Multiple studies have supported that latissimus transfers for external rotation function through active muscular contraction in addition to improving a tenodesis effect. Henseler and colleagues[4] reported that clinically significant improvements in active external rotation with increased latissimus dorsi surface electromyographic activity during activities in shoulder elevation after 12 months of surgery. Porcellini and colleagues[5] similarly reported that external rotation lag signs resolved and increased electromyographic activation of the latissimus dorsi muscle after transfer during active external rotation after a mean follow-up of 16.6 months.

The lower trapezius tendon transfer was introduced by Elhassan and colleagues for treating massive irreparable tears of the posterosuperior cuff after its success in managing shoulder paralysis.[6,7] The trapezius muscle originates from the occiput and the C7-T12 spinous processes, and it consists of 3 parts. The upper trapezius inserts onto the posterior aspect of the distal clavicle. The middle and the lower trapezius both of which insert on the scapular spine. The lower trapezius tendon transfer has a similar line of pull to the infraspinatus, which contracts in phase during external rotation, forward elevation, and abduction. Moreover, the lower trapezius tendon provides better abduction and external rotation moment arms compared with the latissimus tendon transfer. In a cadaveric study by Hartzler and colleagues, the lower trapezius transfer had the highest external rotation moment arm at adduction, and it had the most similar moment to the infraspinatus and teres minor compared with the latissimus tendon transfer.[6] As such, the lower trapezius tendon offers many biomechanical advantages over the latissimus tendon when transferred for deficient posterosuperior rotator cuff.

Muscle tendon transfers for anterosuperior cuff deficiency

Muscle tendon transfer options for reconstructing the anterosuperior rotator cuff (ie, subscapularis and/or supraspinatus), include a latissimus dorsi tendon transfer with or without teres major, or a pectoralis major tendon transfer.

The pectoralis major muscle has 2 portions, the clavicular head and the sternal head. The clavicular head originated from the medial half or two-thirds of the clavicle. The sternal head originated from the sternum and the 2nd to 6th ribs.[8] Both heads insert onto the proximal humerus just lateral to the bicipital groove. The clavicular head mainly assists in shoulder forward flexion, whereas the sternal head mainly contributed to arm adduction and internal rotation. The pectoralis major transfer for the anterosuperior cuff deficiency has the longest track record with numerous variations reported throughout the literature with variable outcomes.[9-12]

The latissimus dorsi tendon transfer is our preferred method for anterosuperior rotator cuff deficiency due to several reasons. The latissimus dorsi muscle is a more appropriate muscle tendon transfer compared with the pectoralis major because its origin is from the posterior chest wall, providing a similar line of pull to the subscapularis muscle. Whereas the pectoralis major muscle originates from an anterior position, which is almost perpendicular to the line of pull of the subscapularis. In our experience, the pectoralis major transfer has failed to resolve preoperative anterior glenohumeral subluxation in the setting of subscapularis deficiency.[12]

Muscle tendon transfers for combined anterior and posterosuperior cuff deficiency

Combined deficiencies of the anterior and posterosuperior cuff present an increasingly challenging issue especially in the young and active individuals. In such patients, our preferred approach is to perform a "Parachute" procedure, which is a combination of a lower trapezius tendon transfer for the posterosuperior cuff and an anterior latissimus dorsi tendon transfer for the subscapularis.[13]

Muscle tendon transfers for deltoid deficiency

The muscle tendon transfer option for deltoid deficiency, especially of the anterior and middle deltoid portions, is a pedicled pectoralis major transfer. The main purpose of this transfer is to restore arm forward elevation through reconstructing the anterior deltoid muscle. The tendon transfer involved detaching the pectoralis major's clavicular portion and the upper half of the sternal head from their origins. Thereafter, the harvested pectoralis major is rotated around its neurovascular pedicle, and then reattached to the lateral clavicle and the anterior acromion. This provides the transferred pectoralis major muscle with a vertical line of pull similar to the anterior deltoid muscle. Another muscle tendon transfer option for deltoid deficiency would be a pedicled latissimus tendon transfer. The main advantage of a pedicled latissimus tendon transfer is providing excellent soft-tissue coverage; however, it provides less strength and range of motions when compared with pedicles pectoralis major transfer.

Rehabilitation After Muscle Tendon Transfer in the Shoulder

Multiple considerations must be considered during shoulder tendon transfer rehabilitation. The patient's preoperative status often predicts the amount of functional improvement after a tendon transfer surgery. This would include preoperative range of motion and the extent of rotator cuff and/or deltoid deficiency. Additionally, one must consider the type of tendon transfer performed. Patient specific demands pertaining to their desired activities and occupation might require tailored rehabilitation program. It is important to match patient expectations according to the aforementioned factors and to focus on gradual improvement.

Rehabilitation after shoulder muscle tendon transfers typically involves 4 phases. The first phase requires appropriate immobilization in an optimal position to ensure muscle–tendon healing with adequate tension. Patients are also educated on brace/cast care, bathing, and cryotherapy. The second phase focuses on initiating active range of motion in a gradual and progressive manner to learn the new muscle activation. The third phase focuses on strengthening and maximizing range of motion. The fourth phase is related to advanced strengthening and to individualize rehabilitation to specific patients' needs and occupation. **Table 1** displays a generic rehabilitation protocol after tendon transfer surgery.

REHABILITATION AFTER MUSCLE TENDON TRANSFER FOR POSTEROSUPERIOR CUFF

Phase 1 entails immobilization and maximal protection of the transferred tendon for 8 weeks. The type of immobilization differs between latissimus tendon transfer and

Table 1
Generic rehabilitation protocol after muscle tendon transfer procedures

Phase	Postoperative Week	Goals	Progression Criteria
I	0–8	Immobilization • External rotation brace for LD transfer for posterosuperior cuff • Shoulder spica cast for pedicled PM transfer for deltoid deficiency • Shoulder abduction brace for all other transfers	Complete 8 wk of immobilization
II	8–16	1. Initiate range of motion • Achieve functional passive range of motion (PROM) and active range of motion (AROM) 2. Transferred tendon retraining	• Achieve pain free AROM • Satisfactory recruitment of the transferred muscle tendon
III	16–24	1. Strengthening: gradual and progressive 2. Achieve maximal range of motion	• Continued satisfactory progress in strength • Continued recruitment of the transferred muscle tendon
IV	≥24	1. Advanced strengthening to restore endurance and strength 2. Return to preferred activities and occupation	• Satisfactory clinical examination • Strength ≥75% of contralateral healthy extremity

the lower trapezius transfer. The latissimus tendon transfer is immobilized in a shoulder brace with an abduction pillow. Whereas the lower trapezius transfer in an external rotation brace at 40° of abduction and 40° of external rotation (**Fig. 1**). The absolute goal of this phase is to protect the integrity of the repair. We advise patients to wear the brace at all times except when performing hygiene, which should be performed with assistance. We also instruct patients to avoid passive internal rotation, adduction, or extension.

Phase 2 occurs from week 8 to week 16, postoperatively, which consists of brace removal and initiating active range of motion. The goal of this phase is (1) to restore functional passive range of motion, (2) to achieve active range of motion with minimal pain, and (3) to retrain the latissimus dorsi or lower trapezius tendon as shoulder external rotator and humeral head depressor. No strengthening or active internal rotation is permitted during this phase. Therapeutic interventions are also permitted such as aqua therapy, biofeedback, and neuromuscular electrical stimulation, which aid in retraining of the transferred muscle tendons. At 12 weeks of phase 2, the internal rotation range of motion limitations are removed.

Phase 3 is focused on strengthening and occurs between 16 and 24 weeks, postoperatively. The main goals of phase 3 are to improve strength and maximize range of motion in a gradual but progressive fashion. Strengthening exercises are started in a supine position to eliminate gravity using bands, and light free weights. Strengthening should focus on all shoulder and periscapular muscles.

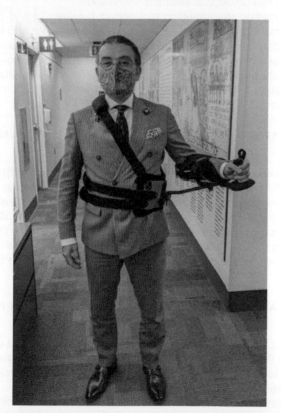

Fig. 1. The external rotation brace typically used after lower trapezius tendon transfer with the arm placed at 40° of abduction and 40° of external rotation.

Phase 4 starts after week 24 and is concerned with advanced strengthening and return to activity. The goals of this stage are to increase endurance and strength of the transferred muscle tendon. Another goal is to enhance neuromuscular control through focusing on advanced closed chain exercises, and proprioception activities such as position awareness and rhythmic stabilization exercises. Patients are permitted to return to their desired activities after a satisfactory physical examination and when strength is achieved at 75% or more compared with the contralateral side.

REHABILITATION AFTER MUSCLE TENDON TRANSFER FOR ANTEROSUPERIOR CUFF

Phase 1 consists of immobilization with a shoulder brace with an abduction pillow for 8 weeks to protect the transferred tendon in an internal rotation position. Patients are educated on brace care, cryotherapy, and advise patients to wear the brace at all times.

Phase 2 occurs between weeks 8 and 16 postoperatively where the brace is removed, and active range of motion is initiated. Two important considerations are to perform shoulder flexion in internal rotation and to refrain from external rotation beyond neutral for 8 weeks. The goal of this phase is to (1) restore functional passive range of motion, (2) to achieve active range of motion with minimal pain, and (3) retrain the latissimus dorsi or pectoralis major tendon as shoulder internal rotator and humeral head depressor. Therapeutic interventions are also permitted such as aqua therapy, biofeedback, and neuromuscular electrical stimulation.

Phase 3 is focused on strengthening and occurs between 16 and 24 weeks, postoperatively. The main goals of phase 3 are to improve strength and maximize range of motion in a gradual but progressive fashion. Phase 4 starts after week 24 and is concerned with advanced strengthening, return to activity, and to enhance neuromuscular control. Patients are permitted to return to their desired activities after a satisfactory physical examination and when strength is achieved at 75% or more compared with the contralateral side.

REHABILITATION AFTER A COMBINED ANTERIOR AND POSTEROSUPERIOR TENDON TRANSFERS

The shoulder is immobilized using an abduction shoulder brace with neutral rotation for an 8-week duration. Between 8 and 16 weeks, rehabilitation is focused on active-assisted range of motion exercises and aqua therapy. At 16-week postoperatively, progressive stretching and strengthening is initiated for another 8 weeks to attain maximum range of motion and strength. Patients may resume their full activities without limitations at 6 months postoperatively after a satisfactory physical examination and when strength is achieved at 75% or more compared with the contralateral side.

REHABILITATION AFTER A PEDICLED PECTORALIS MAJOR TRANSFER FOR DELTOID DEFICIENCY

Phase 1 immobilization consists of shoulder spica cast for a period of 8 weeks. The arm remains in a flexed position of 45° to 60° with neutral rotation to 40° of external rotation, similar to singing into a microphone (**Fig. 2**). After 8 weeks, the brace is removed, and patients are advanced to phase 2.

The second phase of rehabilitation starts between week 8 and week 16 and focuses on initiating gentle passive range of motion, starting active-assisted range of motion and aqua therapy for a total of 8 weeks. The goal of phase 2 is to achieve minimal

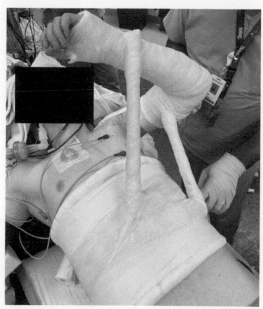

Fig. 2. A shoulder spica cast with the arm position in a flexed position of 45° to 60° with neutral rotation to 40° of external rotation, similar to singing into a microphone.

pain with active range of motion, restore functional passive range of motion, and retrain the transferred pectoralis major as a shoulder flexor.

Phase 3 starts between 16 and 24 weeks, which consists of gentle strengthening and with bands and light free weights starting in supine position and focusing on shoulder elevation. Phase 4 starts at 6 months with activity as tolerated and a weight restriction of 15 lbs in any direction. Gradual, progressive stretching as tolerated can occur at this point and is prohibited before this point to prevent muscle stretch injuries.

SUMMARY

Muscle tendon transfer procedures in the shoulder require a detailed and lengthy rehabilitation to achieve satisfactory outcomes. Surgeons and physical therapists must gain in-depth understanding for each tendon transfer procedure such as immobilization requirements and specific restrictions at each rehabilitation time point. Additionally, one must consider the patient preoperative function and the severity of muscular deficits to manage patients' expectations and focus on gradual but progressive improvement. Individualized therapeutic interventions must be actively implemented to help patients achieve their goals and return to their desired function.

CLINICS CARE POINTS

- Posterosuperior cuff deficiency is treated with a lower trapezius or latissimus dorsi tendon transfer, and it is immobilized for 8 weeks with an external rotation brace.

- Anterosuperior cuff deficiency is treated with an anterior latissimus dorsi transfer or pectoralis major transfer. Subsequently it is immobilized for 8 weeks in a shoulder brace with an abduction pillow.

- If combined muscle transfers for anterior and posterior cuff deficiency is performed, patients should be immobilized for 8 weeks in a shoulder abduction brace in neutral rotation.

- Pedicled pectoralis major transfers are performed for deltoid deficiency and requires immobilization for 8 weeks in a shoulder spica cast with the arm in 40-65° forward flexion, and arm external rotation up to 40°.

- After the immobilization period is completed, patients are advanced through additional three stages consisting of gradual range of motion, strengthening.

DECLARATION OF INTERESTS

The authors have nothing to disclose.

REFERENCES

1. Williams PE, Goldspink G. The effect of immobilization on the longitudinal growth of striated muscle fibres. J Anat 1973;116(Pt 1):45–55.
2. Koh TJ, Herzog W. Increasing the moment arm of the tibialis anterior induces structural and functional adaptation: implications for tendon transfer. J Biomech 1998;31(7):593–9.
3. Takahashi M, Ward SR, Marchuk LL, et al. Asynchronous muscle and tendon adaptation after surgical tensioning procedures. J Bone Joint Surg Am 2010; 92(3):664–74.
4. Henseler JF, Nagels J, Nelissen RG, et al. Does the latissimus dorsi tendon transfer for massive rotator cuff tears remain active postoperatively and restore active external rotation? J Shoulder Elbow Surg 2014;23(4):553–60.
5. Porcellini G, Padolino A, Merolla G, et al. Latissimus Dorsi Tendon Transfer for Irreparable Rotator Cuff Tears: Clinical, EMG and Kinematic Results of Arthroscopically Assisted Approach vs Fully Open Approach. JSES Open Access 2019;3(4):236.
6. Hartzler RU, Barlow JD, An KN, et al. Biomechanical effectiveness of different types of tendon transfers to the shoulder for external rotation. J Shoulder Elbow Surg 2012;21(10):1370–6.
7. Elhassan BT, Wagner ER, Werthel JD. Outcome of lower trapezius transfer to reconstruct massive irreparable posterior-superior rotator cuff tear. J Shoulder Elbow Surg 2016;25(8):1346–53.
8. Fung L, Wong B, Ravichandiran K, et al. Three-dimensional study of pectoralis major muscle and tendon architecture. Clin Anat 2009;22(4):500–8.
9. Wirth MA, Rockwood CA Jr. Operative treatment of irreparable rupture of the subscapularis. J Bone Joint Surg Am 1997;79(5):722–31.
10. Ernstbrunner L, Wieser K, Catanzaro S, et al. Long-Term Outcomes of Pectoralis Major Transfer for the Treatment of Irreparable Subscapularis Tears: Results After a Mean Follow-up of 20 Years. J Bone Joint Surg Am 2019;101(23):2091–100.
11. Resch H, Povacz P, Ritter E, et al. Transfer of the pectoralis major muscle for the treatment of irreparable rupture of the subscapularis tendon. J Bone Joint Surg Am 2000;82(3):372–82.
12. Elhassan B, Ozbaydar M, Massimini D, et al. Transfer of pectoralis major for the treatment of irreparable tears of subscapularis: does it work? J Bone Joint Surg Br 2008;90(8):1059–65.
13. Elhassan BT, Dang KH, Huynh TM. Parachute" technique for combined irreparable subscapularis and posterosuperior rotator cuff tears. Obere Extremität 2021;16(4):286–8.

Remote Patient Monitoring of Postoperative Rehabilitation

Brandon J. Erickson, MD[a,b,c,*], Yousef Shishani, MD[d],
Reuben Gobezie, MD[d]

KEYWORDS

• Range of motion • Artificial intelligence • Telerehab

INTRODUCTION

Shoulder problems are one of the most common ailments seen by orthopedic surgeons. Although many shoulder issues can be managed conservatively, those who fail a trial of conservative treatment are often indicated for operative intervention. Although there are countless types of shoulder surgeries, there is one common thread with almost all patients who undergo a shoulder operation: they require postoperative rehabilitation. The goal of postoperative rehabilitation is initially to protect the surgery while maximizing healing. This is often followed by a several week period to regain shoulder range of motion (ROM). Once shoulder motion has returned, patients are often allowed to strengthen the shoulder. The symbiotic relationship of shoulder surgery and postoperative rehabilitation has produced reliable results following such procedures as rotator cuff repair, labral repair, and shoulder arthroplasty.[1–7]

Although postoperative rehabilitation has historically been performed in person, there has been a recent shift to remote therapy options. This is partly due to the COVID-19 pandemic but has also been driven by patients who have difficulty making the time commitments necessary to get to a therapy location, have their therapy, and then get home or to work. In 2020, Medicare approved the use of real-time face-to-face technology for physical therapists, which allowed therapists to offer both in-person as well as remote rehabilitation options.

[a] Rothman Orthopaedic Institute, 645 Madison Avenue, New York, NY 10022, USA;
[b] Department of Orthopaedic Surgery, Sidney Kimmel Medical College of Thomas Jefferson University; [c] Grossman School of Medicine, New York University; [d] Cleveland Shoulder Institute, 25501 Chagrin Boulevard, Suite 200, Beachwood, OH 44122, USA
* Corresponding author. Rothman Orthopaedic Institute, 645 Madison Avenue, New York, NY 10022.
E-mail address: brandon.erickson@rothmanortho.com

Phys Med Rehabil Clin N Am 34 (2023) 489–497
https://doi.org/10.1016/j.pmr.2022.12.011
1047-9651/23/© 2022 Elsevier Inc. All rights reserved.

Options for Remote Therapy

Although in-person therapy is relatively straightforward, there can be many different types of remote therapy on many different platforms. Remote monitoring of patients can be as simple as a telephone call to try to assess their ROM, strength, and so forth. This is difficult because you are relying on the patients to accurately measure their ROM and strength. A second option is to use an application-based rehabilitation program where the patients follow a designated series of exercises each day, and their compliance with these exercises is monitored by a therapist. These applications can sometimes offer a visual option, whereby the therapist can watch the patient performing their exercises as either a live or a recorded video. This can provide an enhanced level of feedback for the patient because errors in their form can be corrected in relatively short order. Finally, and often times most commonly, physical therapists can spend their session live with the patient over one of the many video conferencing platforms. This will permit the therapist to observe the patient in real time and will allow them to make real-time adjustments to the therapy regimen depending on how patients are responding. It will also allow the therapist to confirm patients are performing their therapy exercises correctly so as to not damage the shoulder.

Benefits to Remote Postoperative Physical Therapy

Many therapists, surgeons, and patients are still learning about all of the benefits of remote physical therapy. Although many unknown benefits may still exist, there are several that have become obvious because more patients have transitioned to remote physical therapy. First, remote physical therapy allows patients who are still worried about coming to in-person therapy because of risks of transmitting COVID-19 or other diseases to still participate in therapy. Although the risk of COVID-19 will wane with time, there may be other events that may threaten the ability of therapists to provide in-person care. As such, a remote option allows therapists to reach those patients who are hesitant to come to in-person rehabilitation. Second, many patients who undergo shoulder surgery, especially shoulder arthroplasty and rotator cuff repair, are often older. Some of these patients no longer drive, and it can be difficult to get them into a therapist's office twice per week for several months. Furthermore, for the first several weeks after shoulder surgery, most surgeons advise against driving. As such, if patients do not have a relative or friend to take them to and from therapy, this can be challenging. A remote physical therapy option solves both problems because it allows patients to participate in physical therapy from home, without having to worry about transportation.

Possible Risks Associated with Postoperative Physical Therapy

Although remote physical therapy has many benefits, there are some potential risks that come with this option. These risks can be broken down into 3 main categories. First, there is a risk that the patient simply does not do the therapy as religiously because they do not have to physically go to a therapist's office. Although the remote option can help therapists stay on top of patients to make sure they are doing their therapy, it is easier for a patient to cancel or miss a remote session than skip an in-person session. Second, there is a risk that patients progress more slowly than usual through their therapy because they do not have someone to push them by physically demonstrating on them that they can do more than they think. Similarly, if the patient does not have hands on physical therapy, it can be hard to really push their passive ROM. Finally, there is a risk that the patients progress too quickly and do more than they should and end up compromising the surgical repair. Some patients will not fully understand the difference between passive and active ROM, or may not understand the necessity to start with lightweights when progressing to strengthening exercises. As such, they may run the risk of compromising their repair.

Current Literature

As telerehab is relatively new, studies reporting outcomes of remote rehabilitation are just beginning to emerge. Although the purpose of this article is to discuss remote rehabilitation for the shoulder, there have been studies evaluating the effectiveness of telerehab for other musculoskeletal problems as well. Beresford and colleagues reported on the results of telerehab for 814 patients, 132 (16%) of whom were performing rehabilitation for their shoulder.[8] The authors noted significant decreases in pain and clinically significant increases in function following virtual rehabilitation. Unfortunately, the authors did not have a control group of patients who went to in-person rehabilitation to compare the results with, so it is unclear if the benefits these patients achieved from telerehab would be similar, worse or better compared with patients going to in-person therapy. One barrier to telerehab that must be discussed is patient perceptions of telerehab compared with in-person rehabilitation. Sabesan and colleagues followed 80 patients who underwent shoulder surgery followed by in-person rehabilitation and asked their perceptions of telerehab.[9] Interestingly, 52.5% of patients surveyed did not think they would be able to achieve successful outcomes with virtual rehabilitation and 68.6% of patients stated they would not consider transitioning to virtual rehabilitation following a few in-person sessions. Hence, there seems to be some perceptions surrounding virtual rehabilitation that need to be addressed before this can be widely accepted.

Gava and colleagues performed a systematic review to report effects of physical therapy performed through telehealth on patients with shoulder pain.[10] They included 6 randomized studies with a total of 368 patients who complained of shoulder pain. The indications for rehabilitation were different across the studies as 3 studies assessed shoulder postoperative care, 2 assessed chronic shoulder pain and 1 assessed patients with frozen shoulder. The studies included in this review were low quality but the results showed that there was no difference between telerehabilitation and in-person physical therapy to improve pain and disability in patients with shoulder pain.

Greiner and colleagues reported the outcomes of 132 patients who underwent at home rehabilitation following shoulder surgery.[11] The authors noted that both pain scores and pain medication use decreased from the first to eighth postoperative telehealth session and that patient satisfaction scores were high. Furthermore, Rennie and colleagues discussed telemedicine rehabilitation for the shoulder as well as the knee and noted there was a cost savings to patients, adding to the benefit of remote rehabilitation.

Interestingly, although rehabilitation has often followed a standard protocol, gamification has emerged as an option for postoperative rehabilitation in shoulder patients.[12] Marley and colleagues performed a randomized controlled trial where they randomized 64 patients who underwent arthroscopic shoulder surgery to either standard in-person physical therapy (n = 31) or remote gamification with exergames (active, gamified video-based exercises) (n = 33).[12] Gamification essentially incorporates game mechanics in a nongame setting using a tailored user interface, which may encourage engagement through rewards, competition, and immediate feedback. The authors found no significant difference in any ROM measurements between groups.

Similarly, there was no difference in the improvement in the Oxford Shoulder Score or Disabilities of the Arm, Shoulder, and Hand score between groups. The authors concluded that remote exergames is a viable treatment option following shoulder surgery.

The Author's Experience with Telerehab

There are many platforms that offer telerehab, and there are advantages and disadvantages of each system. There are several factors to consider including cost, reimbursement, functionality, ease of use, and so forth. Some examples of telerehab platforms include PT Genie (Orlando, FL), ROM Tech (Brookfield, CT), and many others. There are also physical therapy companies that will provide their services through virtual visits. Studies regarding effectiveness of specific platforms are ongoing, and it is still too early to make a firm recommendation on one platform that is superior to others. This may change as telerehab becomes more common and studies gain power by recruiting more and more patients but, for now, the surgeon and patient should use a platform they are familiar with and comfortable with its functionality.

In our practice, which is exclusively a shoulder practice, we have been using PT Genie (Orlando, Fl.) to conduct telerehab and remote patient monitoring. The PT Genie digital platform has 2 modules, a virtual monitored rehab module and a 3-D assessment module.

The technology used in the virtual rehab application is a markerless 2-D artificial intelligence (AI)-powered motion capture that can be used on both iOS and Android devices (**Fig. 1**). When the application is downloaded onto a patient's device, it can

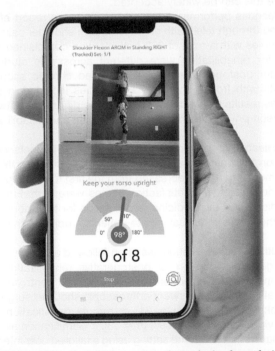

Fig. 1. AI-powered technology that tracks motion through the front-facing camera. (*From PT Genie;* https://genie.health/pt-genie/.)

provide custom physical therapy protocols with monitored and tracked exercises for all major joints (*neck*, *back*, *shoulder*, *elbow*, *wrist*, *hip*, *knee*, *ankle*). Through the front-facing camera of a mobile device, PT Genie gives instant corrective feedback as the patients perform their home-based exercises and provides monitoring of daily progress. The data from the patient's application is securely and instantly pushed to the provider web portal for easy access and visualization. The platform also includes a telemedicine component that enables secure video calls between the provider and the patient that is designed to be user-friendly, efficient, and convenient (**Fig. 2**). In our practice, we offer the PT Genie rehab pathway to all our patients as an adjunct to traditional in-office physical therapy. This "hybrid" approach has many benefits such as the following: (1) increase the case load for our PT department, (2) patients reporting higher satisfaction with their recovery, and (3) increase the percent of scheduled PT televisits and the overall engagement on the digital platform. Interestingly in our practice, when we examined engagement on the digital platform, we observed that it was highest in older patients undergoing a shoulder arthroplasty procedure. Patients aged between 51 and 70 years completed more than 70% of the prescribed rehab sessions (**Fig. 3**). This fortified our day-to-day observations that such technology is not a barrier for the elderly patient.

The PT Genie 3D assessment module is built on more advanced algorithms and uses the LiDAR scanner, which is found on portable devices such as an iPad pro. This technology enables the health-care provider to analyze and measure complex multijoint motions in less than 5 minutes, producing a large amount of data that is instantly translated into a variety of applications, including but not limited to: Advanced movement screening and injury prevention, workplace wellness, gait analysis, balance, and posture testing (**Fig. 4**).

From the Patient's Perspective

The patient/mobile facing PT Genie application was designed to be used by virtually anyone who owns a smartphone. The application is available on both the Apple and Google app stores, and with a simple scan to a custom QR code the application is downloaded immediately onto the patient's smartphone/tablet (**Fig. 5**). The user does not need any additional hardware to perform the home-based rehab exercises. A dedicated PT Genie team ensures that the patient is "virtually" hand-held throughout

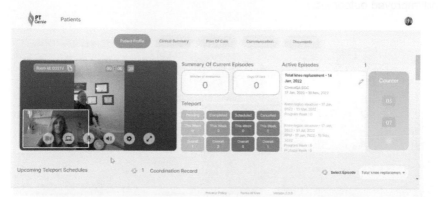

Fig. 2. The built-in telemedicine platform enables both parties to interact in a secure, fast, and efficient environment. (*From PT Genie;* https://genie.health/pt-genie/.)

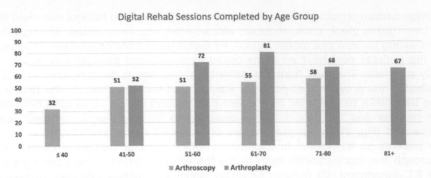

Fig. 3. The highest engagement was observed in older patients undergoing shoulder arthroplasty procedures.

the rehab journey, from downloading the app to completing a fully custom rehab program. The PT Genie platform enables a 2-way communication between the patient and the care provider, which ultimately helps the patient recover under the close observation of the care team. This turnkey process is continuously updated, optimized, and perfected to make the user-experience as smooth and seamless as possible.

From the Surgeon's Perspective

The provider-facing portal in PT Genie is a secure, web-based instance that can be accessed from any computer. The provider portal communicates with the patient-facing application and displays all pertinent information regarding the recovery of the patient. PT Genie allows immediate access and visualization of relevant outcomes that were previously remotely unavailable. By accessing the patient's profile, we are now able to monitor and track the patient's progress, and instantly modify the rehab plan of care, if needed. A clinical dashboard displays pain scores visual analog scale (VAS) and multiple joints ranges of motion trends, as well as exercise compliance tracking (**Fig. 6**). Secure messaging and video calls allow direct interactions between the patient and the health-care provider, which helps in remotely managing the patient's progress and continuity of care. Using such technologies and digital tools in our practice led to a positive impact regarding patient engagement, quality of care, and improved outcomes.

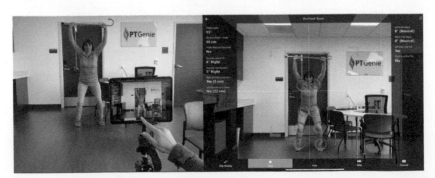

Fig. 4. An iPad pro running the 3-dimensional advanced screening application. (*From PT Genie;* https://genie.health/pt-genie/.)

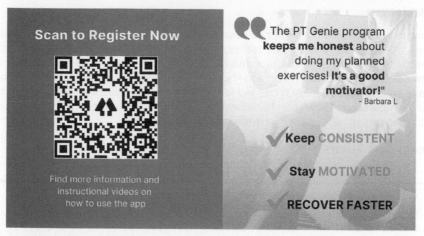

Fig. 5. Custom QR code handouts are used to facilitate the onboarding process. (*From* PT Genie; https://genie.health/pt-genie/.)

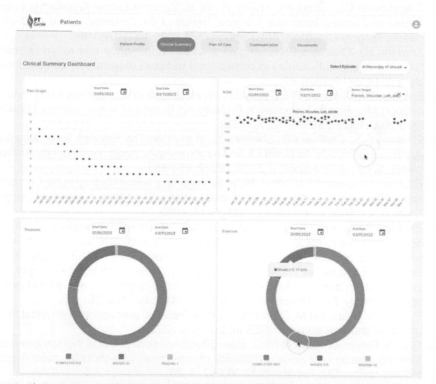

Fig. 6. The provider dashboard showing pain score and ROM tracking as well as compliance charts. (*From PT Genie;* https://genie.health/pt-genie/.)

SUMMARY

Remote rehabilitation following shoulder surgery has become a viable option for patients. Although there are some procedures that may be more amenable to virtual rehabilitation such as biceps tenodesis, distal clavicle excision, and so forth than others such as rotator cuff repair and shoulder arthroplasty, the need for a remote option is critical. Further study is needed to directly compare results of virtual rehabilitation to in-person rehabilitation to determine if there is a difference in outcomes, or if both methods of rehabilitation provide equivalent outcomes.

CLINICS CARE POINTS

- Virtual Rehabilitation is becoming more and more common.
- Surgeons must adapt to incorporate virtual rehabilitation into their repertoire to best serve their patients and ensure optimal outcomes.

REFERENCES

1. Cabarcas BC, Gowd AK, Liu JN, et al. Establishing maximum medical improvement following reverse total shoulder arthroplasty for rotator cuff deficiency. J Shoulder Elbow Surg 2018;27(9):1721-31.
2. Cvetanovich GL, Gowd AK, Frantz TL, et al. Superior Labral Anterior Posterior Repair and Biceps Tenodesis Surgery: Trends of the American Board of Orthopaedic Surgery Database. Am J Sports Med 2020;48(7):1583-9.
3. Erickson BJ, Chalmers PN, D'Angelo J, et al. Performance and return to sport following rotator cuff surgery in professional baseball players. J Shoulder Elbow Surg 2019;28(12):2326-33.
4. Erickson BJ, Chalmers PN, D'Angelo J, et al. Update on Performance and Return to Sport After Biceps Tenodesis in Professional Baseball Players. Orthop J Sports Med 2022;10(2). 23259671221074732.
5. Erickson B.J., Chalmers P., Shishani Y., et al., Can The Reverse Total Shoulder Arthroplasty Provide As Good Of An Outcome As An Anatomic Shoulder Arthroplasty, Semin In Arthroplasty, 32 (4), 2022, 850-855.
6. Erickson BJ, Denard PJ, Griffin JW, et al. Initial and 1-Year Radiographic Comparison of Reverse Total Shoulder Arthroplasty With a Short Versus Standard Length Stem. J Am Acad Orthop Surg 2022;30(14):e968-78.
7. Erickson BJ, Werner BC, Griffin JW, et al. A comprehensive evaluation of the association of radiographic measures of lateralization on clinical outcomes following reverse total shoulder arthroplasty. J Shoulder Elbow Surg 2021;31(5):963-70.
8. Beresford L, Norwood T. Can physical therapy deliver clinically meaningful improvements in pain and function through a mobile app? an observational retrospective study. Arch Rehabil Res Clin Transl 2022;4(2):100186.
9. Sabesan VJ, Dawoud M, Stephens BJ, et al. Patients' perception of physical therapy after shoulder surgery. JSES Int 2022;6(2):292-6.
10. Gava V, Ribeiro LP, Barreto RPG, et al. Effectiveness of physical therapy given by telerehabilitation on pain and disability of individuals with shoulder pain: A systematic review. Clin Rehabil 2022;36(6):715-25.
11. Greiner JJ, Drain NP, Lesniak BP, et al. Self-Reported Outcomes in Early Postoperative Management After Shoulder Surgery Using a Home-Based Strengthening

and Stabilization System With Telehealth. Sports Health 2022. 1941738122111 6319.

12. Marley WD, Barratt A, Pigott T, et al. A multicenter randomized controlled trial comparing gamification with remote monitoring against standard rehabilitation for patients after arthroscopic shoulder surgery. J Shoulder Elbow Surg 2022; 31(1):8–16.

Moving?

Make sure your subscription moves with you!

To notify us of your new address, find your **Clinics Account Number** (located on your mailing label above your name), and contact customer service at:

Email: journalscustomerservice-usa@elsevier.com

800-654-2452 (subscribers in the U.S. & Canada)
314-447-8871 (subscribers outside of the U.S. & Canada)

Fax number: 314-447-8029

Elsevier Health Sciences Division
Subscription Customer Service
3251 Riverport Lane
Maryland Heights, MO 63043

*To ensure uninterrupted delivery of your subscription, please notify us at least 4 weeks in advance of move.

Printed and bound by CPI Group (UK) Ltd, Croydon, CR0 4YY

13/10/2024

01773494-0001